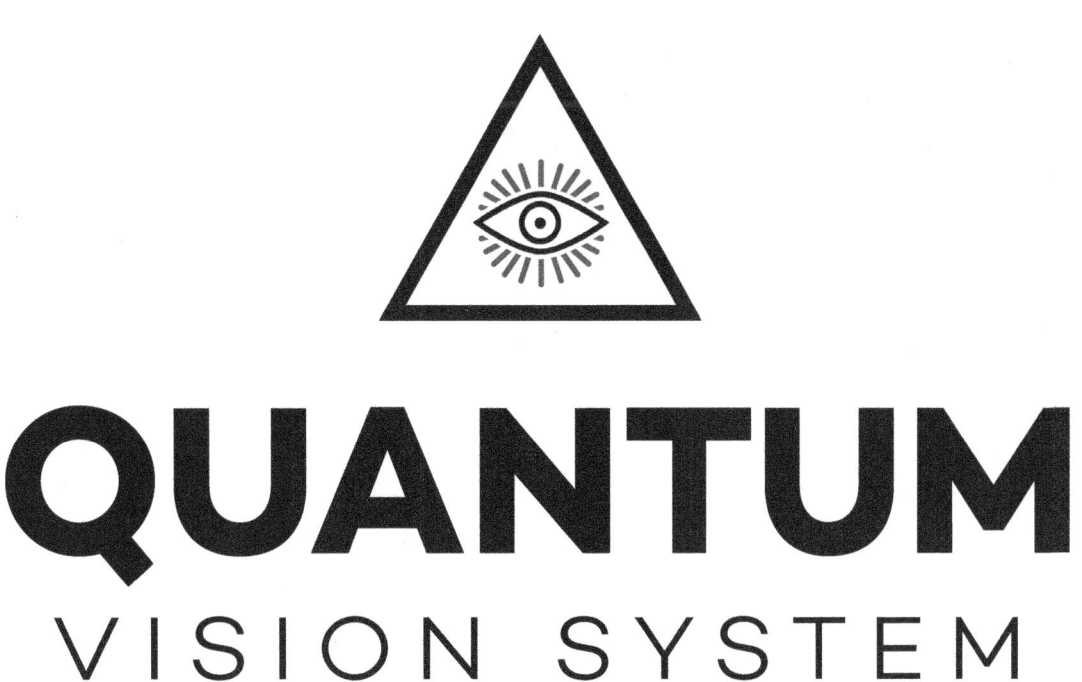

QUANTUM
VISION SYSTEM

Restoring Vision At The Speed Of Light

Legal Disclaimer

The contents of this document are based upon my opinions of the Quantum Vision System, unless otherwise noted. This work is intended to share knowledge and information learned through research, experience, and discussions with others. The opinions of others, such as in the comments and the forum, are their own and are not endorsed by the Quantum Vision System.

The information contained herein is not intended to diagnose, treat, cure or prevent any condition or disease, but rather to provide general information that is intended to be used for educational purposes only. Please consult with your physician or health care practitioner if you have any concerns.

By using, viewing and interacting with the Quantum Vision System or the *QuantumVision System.com* website, you agree to all terms of engagement, thus assuming complete responsibility for your own actions. The authors and publishers will not claim accountability, nor shall they be held liable for any loss or injury sustained by you. Use, view and interact with these resources at your own risk.

All products and information given to you by Quantum Vision System and its related companies are strictly for informational purposes only. While every attempt has been made to verify the accuracy of information provided on our website and within our publications, neither the authors nor the publishers are responsible for assuming liability for possible inaccuracies.

The authors and publishers disclaim any responsibility for the inaccuracy of the content, including but not limited to errors or omissions. Loss of property, injury to self or others, and even death could occur as a direct or indirect consequence of the use and application of any content found herein. Please act responsibly.

The information provided may need to be downloaded and/or viewed using third party software, such as Acrobat or Flash Player. It's the user's responsibility to install the software necessary to view such information. Any downloads, whether purchased or given for free from our website, related websites or hosting systems are performed at the user's own risk. Although we take great preventative measures, we cannot warranty that our websites are free of corrupting computer codes, viruses or worms.

If you are a minor, you can use this service only with permission and guidance from your parents or guardians. Children are not eligible to use our services unsupervised. Furthermore, our website specifically denies access to any individual covered by the Child Online Privacy Act (COPA) of 1998.

Contents

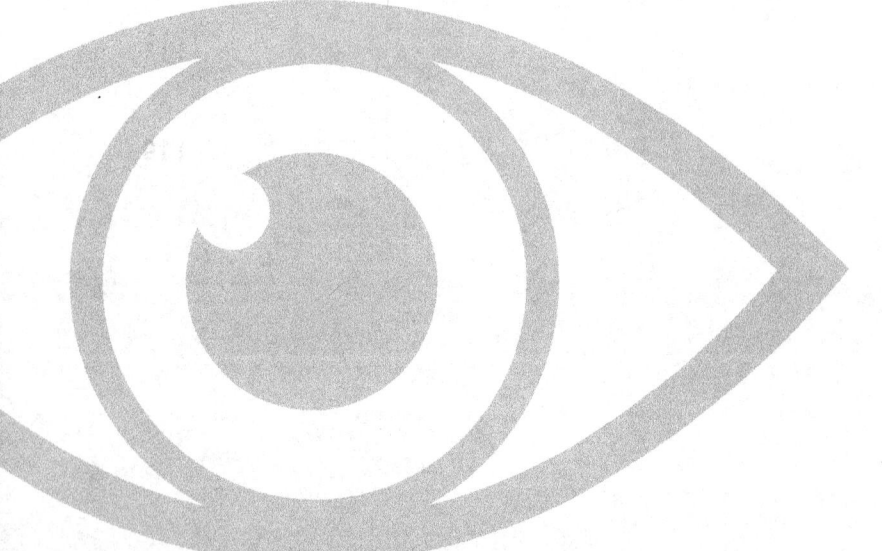

PART 1
VISION
DECEPTION

CHAPTER 1

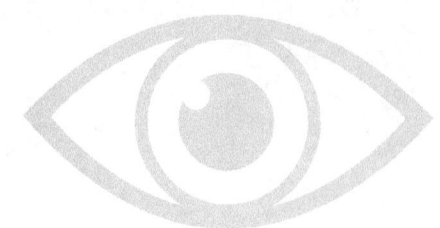

INTRODUCTION

Welcome to the Quantum Vision System. You've taken a big step in becoming glasses free. I'm sure you're just as excited as I am to throw away your glasses and contact lenses for good and finally be able to spend your hard earned money on something besides correcting your vision.

If you read this book and do what it says, I promise you will restore your vision back to 20/20 in just days.

Now I don't believe in miracles, I've done my research and I know what works and what doesn't. Quantum Vision System is based on the groundbreaking work of William Bates, which allows you to restore vision naturally, without glasses, contact lenses or surgery.

We've taken the best of what William Bates discovered and made if even more powerful, while at the same time making it easier to follow so you get the results you deserve.

I've broken everything down to a simple 3-step process that you'll soon learn. I've also listed specific eye conditions and the exact exercise you'll need to correct your vision.

So, what do you have to lose? Nothing … besides your glasses of course! Everything is backed by our 60-day money back guarantee. If you don't improve your vision or are not 100% satisfied with anything in this book, you can simply let us know and we'll refund your entire purchase, no questions asked.

All we ask is that once you start seeing results, you share your testimonial with the world. Send us a quick email or video letting us know your progress and how Quantum Vision System has helped restore your vision.

My team and I are always here to help you. You can email support at any time with questions, concerns or testimonials to *support@quantumvisionsys.com*.

I can't wait to hear about your success story. I can't wait to see your smiling face as you tell us, for the first time ever you were able to throw away your glasses for good!

So what are you waiting for? Let's get you started on the Quantum Vision System.

CHAPTER 2

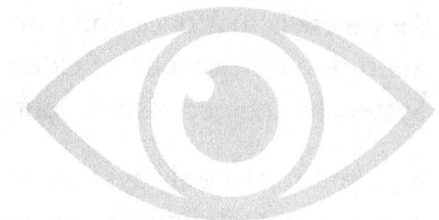

POOR VISION A GROWING PROBLEM

Your eyes are your window to the world. Without your eyes you wouldn't be able to see the sun rise in the morning or set at night, or see the happy faces of your friends and family. Your eyes allow you to experience the world in which you live, that's why you need to do everything you can to keep your vision perfect. Unfortunately, things aren't looking good.

Scary Statistics

In just the last 100 years, eyesight in developed countries has become significantly worse. The numbers for myopia, for example, have gone from 3% of the population to a staggering 42%. And sadly, children appear to be the hardest hit.

Myopia Statistics

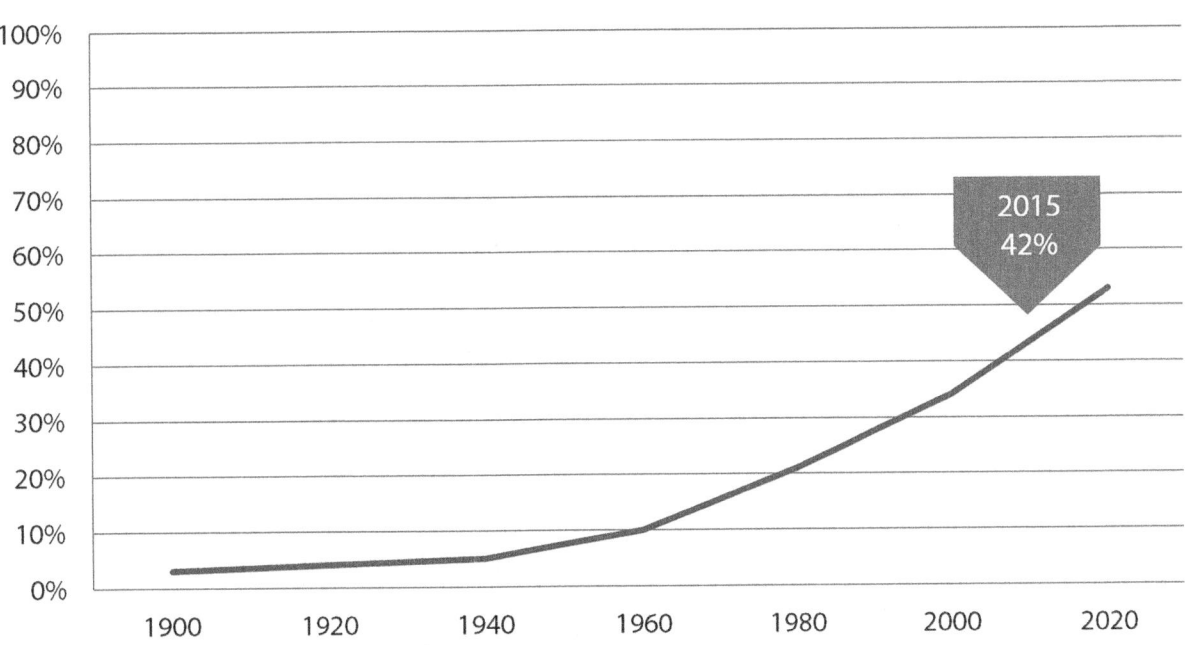

Generally, eye problems get worse with age as seen in the chart below.

2010 U.S. Prevalence Rates Low Vision

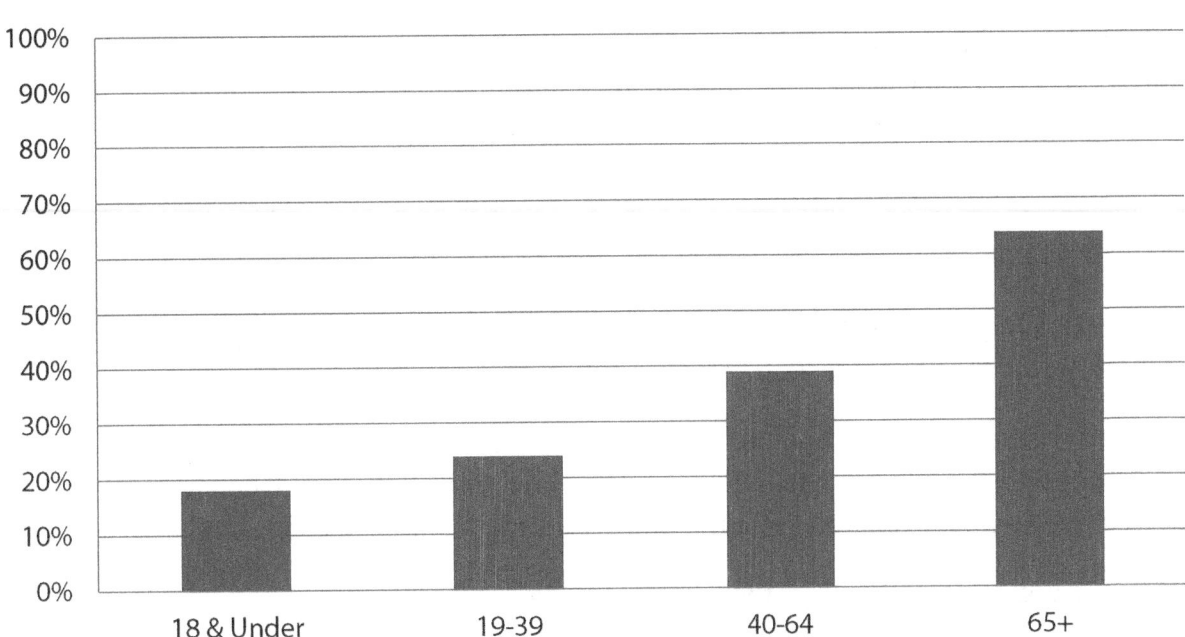

It's also interesting to note the differences between genders. As you can see below, women are much more affected with poor vision.

2010 U.S. Prevalence Rates Low Vision

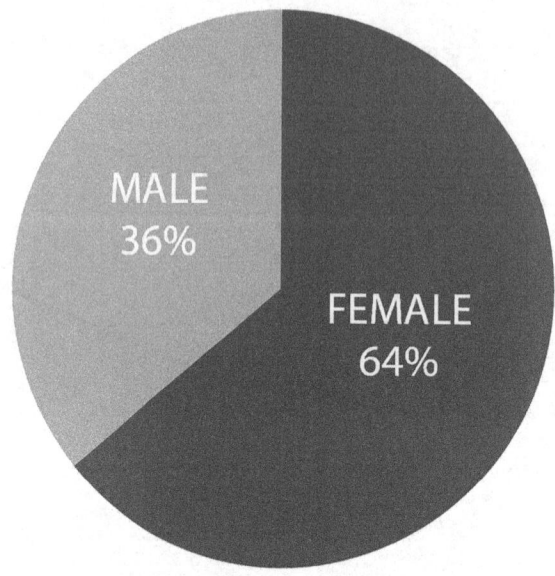

MALE 36%

FEMALE 64%

Later in this book you will learn why eyesight for so many people has gotten so bad, so quickly.

All this data is especially concerning when you consider how important your eyes are. I would bet money that your sense of sight is the most important sense to you. But how exactly do your eyes see everything?

How Your Eyes Work

Your eyes are approximately one inch in diameter and made up of tiny living cells. They contain 70% of the sense receptors in your body.

Protecting the eye are the bones of the skull and pads of fat. The eye is made up of several components – the cornea, pupil, iris, lens, sclera and retina. These components work together to capture an image and send it to the brain through the optic nerve.

Here is a breakdown of each of the eye's components:

Cornea is the front of the eye, which is filled with transparent cells. It acts as a window, allowing light to enter.

Pupil is the dark hole located in the center of the iris. The pupil will become larger or smaller as the iris expands or contracts.

Iris is just behind the cornea. It is a thin circular structure of color muscles, which is responsible for controlling the amount of light that enters through the cornea. The color of the iris is what gives your eye its color.

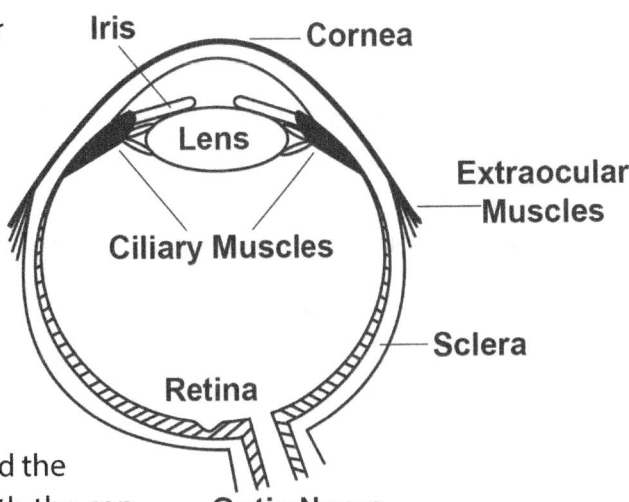

Lens (Inner Lens) is located directly behind the iris. It is a transparent structure of cells with the consistency of rubber that along with the cornea helps focus light onto the retina. The lens can change its shape with the use of Ciliary Muscles, which changes the focal distance of the eye, making it possible to focus on objects at different distances.

Sclera is the white of the eye. It is opaque and contains collagen and elastic fiber. It is considered the protective outer layer of the eye.

Retina is a light-sensitive layer of tissue, which lines the inner surface of the eye. The light that is reflected in from the cornea and lens create an image on the retina. When the light hits the retina it sends chemical and electrical messages that create nerve impulses. These nerve impulses are sent to various visual centers in the brain through the optic nerve fibers at the back of the eye.

Optic Nerve is located at the back of the eye. It transmits the electrical impulses from the retina to the brain. Ultimately it tells our brain what we are looking at.

Extraocular Muscles surround each eyeball. They are in charge of moving the eyes so that both eyes are looking at the same object at the same time.

Did you know that the image that your eye sees is actually upside down?

It's true. When we look at an object in the world, light is reflected off the object and enters through the eye.

Once it enters the eye it becomes altered or distorted. The retina creates a focused, but upside-down image of the object, which is then sent to the brain through the optic nerve. Once the brain receives the image, it then restores the image back to its correct direction while also creating the object to be three-dimensional. Your brain is a powerful thing!

Common Types of Eye Problems

There are several problems that occur specifically within the eye. The list is quite long, considering how small the eye is in our body. But just think of all the components that have to come together to create clear, perfect vision. It's no wonder that approximately 170 million people in the United States need some sort of vision correction.

Below are common eye problems that can occur and their symptoms. Later in this book, we will go into what causes these eye problems and what exercises should be used to help correct the problem.

Nearsightedness (Myopia) – Blurred vision that is worse when looking at distant objects. Often people who have nearsightedness have very good near vision.

Farsightedness (Hyperopia) – Blurred vision when looking at near objects. Sometimes farsightedness is associated with people who have blurred vision to near and far objects.

Astigmatism – Blurry vision at any distance, along with other vision problems.

Retinal Detachment – A condition where the retina pulls away from the support tissue. Symptoms include: A sudden onset of flashing lights often with black floating spots. Sometimes seems like a dark veil or curtain is blocking your vision.

Color Blindness – Difficulty seeing the differences between shades or intensity of color under normal lighting conditions. Usually caused by error in development in one or more sets of the retinal cones that identify color in light and transmit it to the optic nerve. This condition is usually only found in testing for the condition and is mostly found in males.

Night Blindness (Nyctalopia) – Difficulty seeing objects in dim light. Night blindness occurs when the rod cells in the retina slowly lose their ability to react to light.

Cataract – Decreased vision due to clouding of the lens inside the eye, caused by a buildup of yellow-brown pigment on the lens. Symptoms are usually slow to show themselves. Symptoms include: Hazy vision that is worse at night, uncomfortable glare from headlights or bright sunlight, a need for bright light while reading, seeing colors that appear yellow or fading, a milky white appearance to the pupil, painful pressure within the eye and/or double/triple vision in one eye.

Glaucoma – Often when fluid in the eye isn't circulating normally, fluid builds up and causes

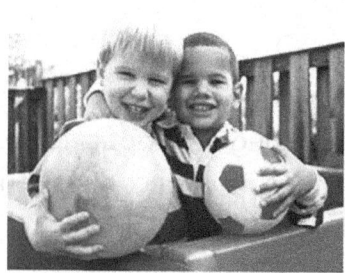

Normal Vision

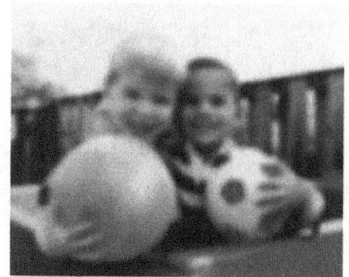

Cataract Vision

increased pressure within the eye. There are two main types of glaucoma – Open-angle and Angle-closure.

» **Open-angle glaucoma** is the most common type. The structure of the eyes appear normal, but fluid does not flow properly through the eye.

» **Angle-closure glaucoma** is less common and can cause sudden buildup of pressure in the eye. Caused by a narrow angled drainage canal between the iris and the cornea.

Symptoms are usually few and the first sign is often the loss of side or peripheral vision.

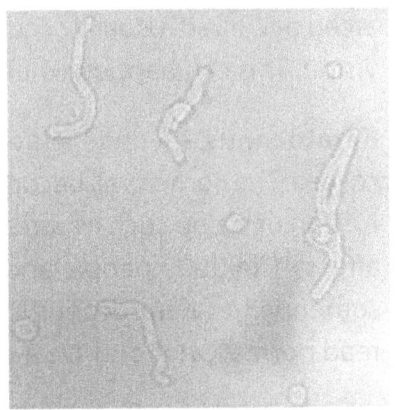

Eye Floaters – Tiny black or gray specks or lines that float into your vision. They should not cause any discomfort or pain. They are usually caused by a natural change in the body of the eye (vitreous humor).

Dry Eye – Eye is unable to produce enough tears to maintain a normal fluid layer to coat your eyes. Without the ability to produce tears, dust or foreign bodies can get into your eye, which can't be disposed of naturally through tears. Symptoms include: stinging, burning, and redness in your eyes.

Strabismus (Heterotropia or Crossed Eyes) – Eyes are not aligned properly, or don't move together. Usually caused by lack of coordination between the extraocular muscles. Eyes could be crossed inwards or outwards. Usually young children with this condition will rub one or both eyes frequently, close one eye to see better or may squint.

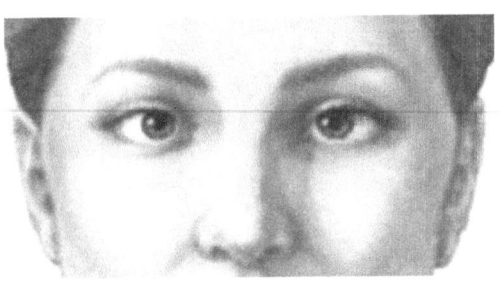

Amblyopia (Lazy Eye) – Eyes are misaligned. Usually one eye is turned in or out. Lazy eye disorder affects 1 – 5% of the world's population.

Occurs when the brain does not fully acknowledge the images it receives from the optic nerve in one of its eyes. Most often occurs in infants during the first few months of life – where development of the optic nerve and brain signals are in affect and hasn't developed properly.

Macular Degeneration – Loss of vision in the center of the visual fields, which is caused by damage to the retina. There are two forms of Macular degeneration – dry and wet.

» **Dry Macular Degeneration** is caused by cellular debris accumulating between the retina and the choroid.

» **Wet Macular Degeneration** is caused by blood vessel growth from the choroid behind the retina.

Both forms can cause the retina to become detached. Symptoms include: gradual, painless loss in central vision, blank spots in your central vision, straight lines appear crooked, and distorted vision while reading.

EpiRetinal Membrane (Macular Pucker) – Disease of the eye caused by changes in the vitreous humor (the fluid in the middle of the eyeball), or diabetes. Often people with EpiRetinal Membrane (or Macular Pucker) will complain about distortion of vision. Lines may appear arced or curved. Usually occurs in one eye first, which can cause binocular diplopia or double vision. This can happen when there is a drastic difference in what each eye sees.

Keratoconus – A degenerative disorder of the eye, which causes structural changes to the cornea. The cornea will become thin and change to a conical shape. This condition causes distortion of vision such as: streaking and sensitivity to light and multiple images. Keratoconus affects 1 in 2000 people and is usually diagnosed in late childhood or early adulthood. If someone has Keratoconus in both eyes, their vision can be so bad that they are unable to read normal print or drive a car.

Later in this book we'll go into detail about the real factors that cause poor vision and what exercises you can do to help cure your eye problem.

In the next chapter we'll talk about how the medical industry is sucking money out of your pocket, and actually causing your eyes to get worse not better!

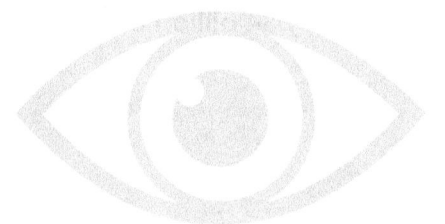

CHAPTER 3

THE VISION INDUSTRY CONSPIRACY

Current Treatment Fraud

What I'm about to tell you might shock you, but it's true. The eye industry has been lying to you for years, blaming genetics for your poor eyesight and claiming there's nothing you can do about it. They don't want you to know that you can easily fix your eyesight and here's why.

Just think about it for a second.

How much money are you spending every year on eye care expenses, going to the eye doctor, picking up prescription glasses, contact lenses and solution? And is your vision getting any better?

Of course not! If you're like most people your eyesight is actually getting worse. And while you suffer, the eye care industry is getting rich.

Every year since 2009 the amount of eyewear sold throughout the United States has increased. In 2012, approximately 18 billion prescription eyeglasses were sold in the U.S.

As most of you know, you are not just paying once for your prescription eyeglasses, you are paying for the lenses, the frames, plus a reflective lens fee and a protection fee. That's on top of your eye doctor visits and any prescriptions they give you. And as you age, your prescription needs become more complicated and it's not uncommon to have a pair of glasses that cost $1000 or more!

The amount of money we spend on eye care is continuingly rising, with no end in sight. Check out the chart below. In 2012, approximately $8.5 billion was spent in the U.S. just on frames, and $10.4 billion on lenses. Americans are spending an enormous amount of money on their eyes. And that doesn't include contact lenses or laser eye surgery, which has been on the rise since the early 2000. In 2012, Americans spent approximately $4 billion on contact lenses and $2 billion on refractive surgery.

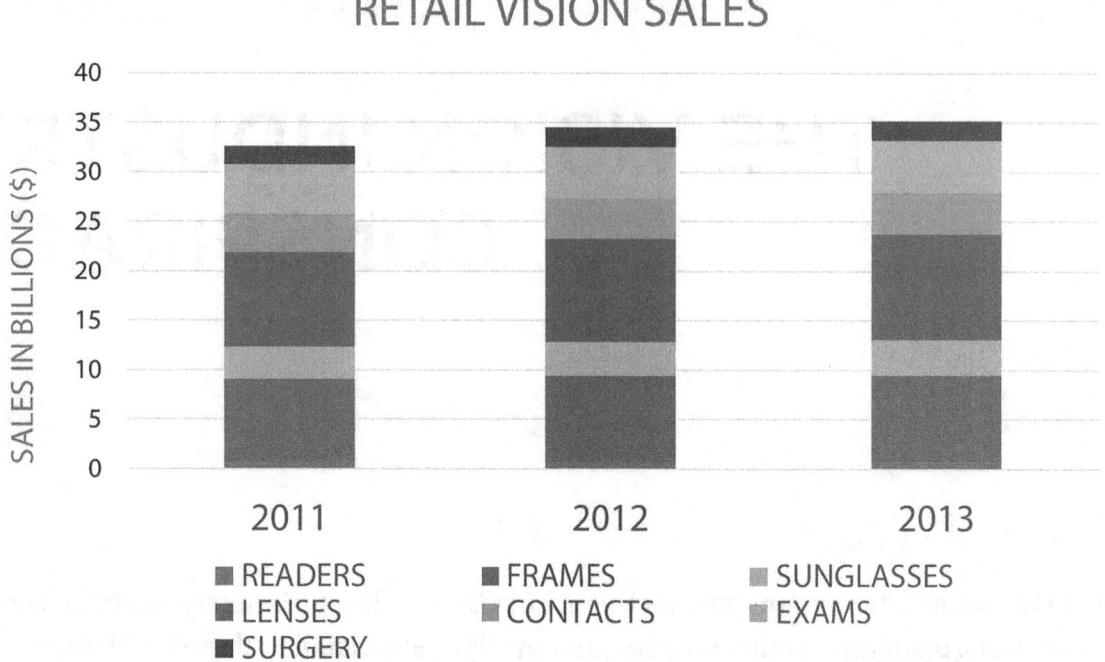

So if eyeglasses and contact lenses aren't helping our vision, why are we wasting all this money? Let's dig into what is really happening to our eyes, since we've become dependent on eyewear.

What Glasses Do To Your Eyes

Your vision is constantly changing. The most common example for this would be how your eyes feel tired after a long day of working at the computer or, how, when you wake up in the morning, it takes you awhile for your eyes to focus.

What eyeglasses are supposed to do is correct the refraction error in our eye, meaning the lens in our glasses is there to reflect the image we see perfectly onto the retina.

Well since we all know lenses aren't flexible, the glasses actually force our vision to stay constantly at that refraction error. Otherwise we wouldn't be able to see through them.

Now what if you had your eyes tested after a long day at the office? Wouldn't your refraction error be worse than it normally is?

That means the glasses you were prescribed are technically causing your eyes to become worse, or become comfortable being in a worse state.

Every time you wear your glasses, especially if you are dependent on your glasses all day (say with astigmatism), your eyes are forced to degrade to the vision level on your glasses just so you can see properly all day. You've probably heard the doctor say "you will get used to your new glasses in a few days".

This is because your eyes are constantly changing and the glasses you were prescribed were for a time when your vision was a little or a lot different than they are when you finally got your glasses.

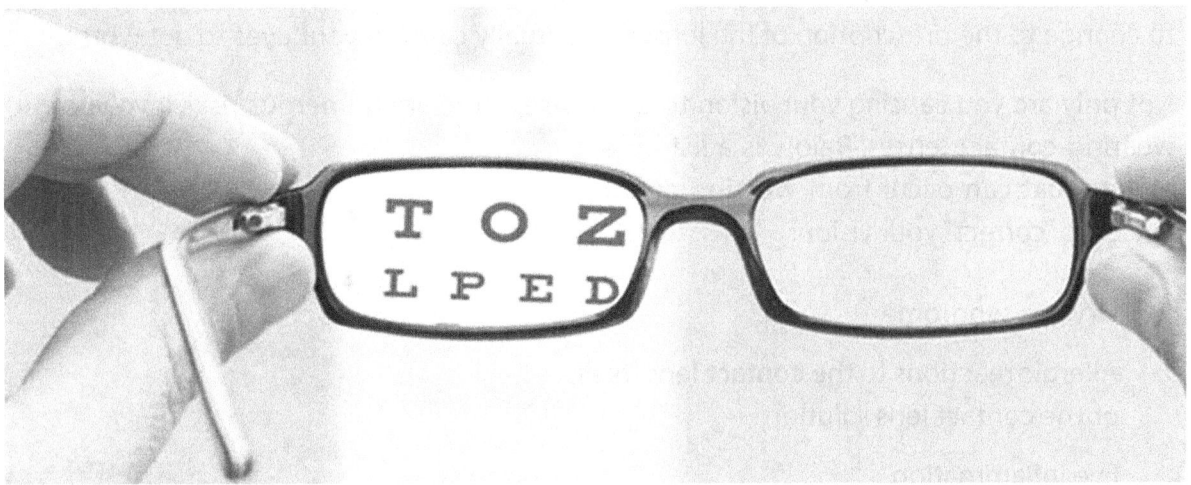

Another reason your eyes require time to "adjust", is because your glasses sit away from your eyes. Your eye now has to change its vision from the space between the glass lens to your eye, and from the object you are focusing on through the lens to your eye.

Your eye is now working double time. This not only affects your vision, it's also an added strain to your eye!

Furthermore, people who are nearsighted, and wear glasses all day cause their eyes to work harder when they focus on objects up-close like a book.

This is because the prescription for the glasses was to correct the refraction error for the person's nearsightedness. So if you are wearing glasses for nearsightedness and want to read a book, you look down through your glasses.

This strains your eyes to focus through a higher prescription and usually around the edge of your frames, which is where the lens bend a bit, so the lens itself isn't even clear.

Your eyes and mind want you to see perfectly so they will adapt to this "new prescription" making your near vision worse.

Scary to think, that your glasses are causing your eyes to be worse, but in all honesty they really are!

What Contact Lenses Do To Your Eyes

Contact lenses are small plastic or silicone discs shaped to correct your refraction error. They are placed directly on your cornea, where they float on a thin layer of tears. Now although improvements have been made in contact lenses, there is still an adjustment period, similar to that of wearing glasses for the first time.

Since your vision constantly changes (as described above), the fact that you cannot easily remove the contact lenses throughout the day, to give your eyes a break causes your eyes to change to the prescription of the lenses, eventually causing your eyes to get worse.

Not only are you causing your vision to get worse, there are numerous risks involved with wearing contact lenses. Below is a list of side effects that can occur from wearing contact lenses to "correct" your vision:

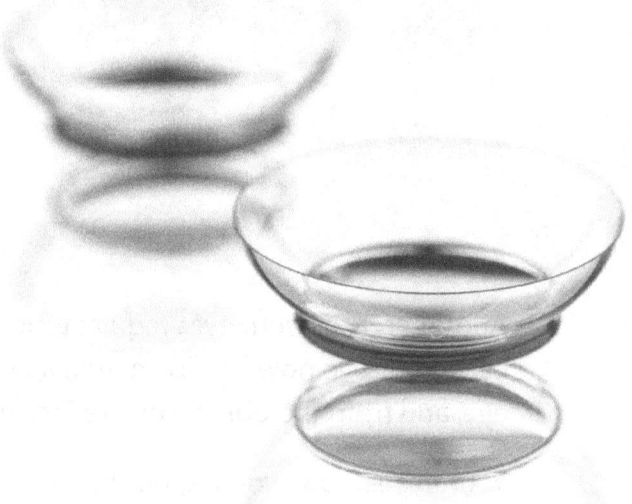

» Dry eye syndrome

» Allergic reactions to the contact lens itself, or the contact lens solution

» Eye inflammation

» Cornea problems:

- Decreased oxygen to the cornea causing swelling and hazy vision

- Scratches on the cornea

- Change in the shape of the cornea

- Infection of the cornea

» Infection due to deposits on the contact lens

» Eyelid inflammation – small bumps under the eyelid

Not to mention the cost. If you regularly use contact lenses, you are looking at paying around $250 per year. Also consider the fact that you likely also own glasses that cost you a pretty penny.

What Laser Eye Surgery Does To Your Eyes

Laser eye surgery is becoming more and more common, but what exactly is this surgery doing to our eyes. Most of our eye problems are caused by an error in the way the eye reflects an image onto the retina, and usually this error occurs because of the cornea's shape. Laser eye surgery consists of a surgeon using a laser device to make permanent changes to the shape of the cornea, which in turn can correct refraction errors in most eyes.

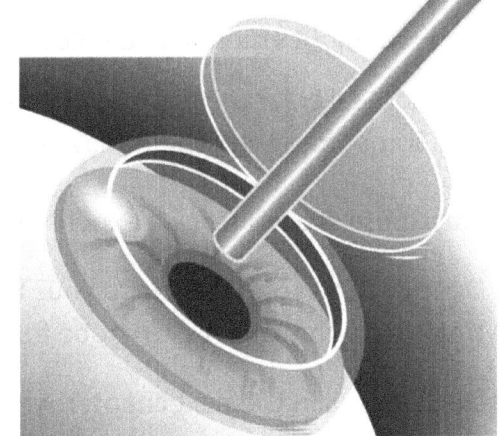

There are several different procedures of laser eye surgery. Below is a breakdown of the different procedures commonly used:

PRK: During surgery the outer layer of the cornea is removed. The laser beam, which is guided by a computer, is used to vaporize tiny amounts of tissue on the cornea. The laser beam is designed to remove the right amount of layers to ultimately change the refraction error in the eye. Usually the healing process is about 1 – 2 weeks.

LASIK: This surgery is more complicated. During surgery the surgeon must first cut a flap in the cornea with a blade or a laser, lifting away from the top of the cornea. Then using the same technique as PRK, a computer-guided laser removes layers of the cornea to change the refraction error of the eye.

The flap is then replaced over the changed cornea. The recovery period is usually much quicker than PRK, approximately 3 – 4 days.

Now, not only have you permanently changed your eyes, there are some side effects that can occur when getting laser eye surgery done. Below is a list of the side effects and risks involved:

PRK risks

» Pain for the first few days after surgery

» Hazy vision while the eyes are healing (usually clears up within a week, sometimes is permanent)

» Regression in vision – sometimes the eye regresses back to the previous refraction error within six months of the surgery. If this happens the patient may have to return for more surgery or will have to return to wearing glasses or contact lenses.

LASIK risks

» Dry eye syndrome – sometimes it can affect the vision of the eye

» Poor night vision due to halos or glare

» Corneal ectasia – a serious condition which is the bulging and weakening of the cornea. Sometimes the patient may need to be treated with a corneal transplant or implant.

Plus, these procedures are expensive, and can set you back up to $10,000.

Does this all sound terrible to you? Your hard earned money is being spent on devices and treatments that aren't even good for you (or really necessary, for that matter).

Don't worry, in the next chapter, we'll show you exactly why your vision gets bad. Later in the book we'll show you exactly what you can do to restore your vision to 20/20.

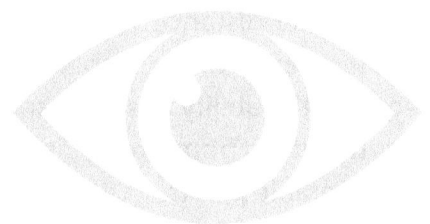

CHAPTER 4
THE TRUE CAUSE OF BAD VISION

Why Your Vision Gets Bad

Although most doctors will say that poor eyesight is the results of genetics, this just isn't true.

Humans have evolved to have excellent vision. In hunter-gatherer days, our ancestors depended upon good vision for survival. If you can't see well enough to decipher the outline of a hungry predator watching you, you're probably not going to make it very long.

Likewise, if your vision doesn't allow you to participate effectively in either hunting or foraging expeditions, your chances are likewise diminished. Although you might have survived young childhood under the watchful eye of tribal caretakers, you probably wouldn't have made it long enough to procreate.

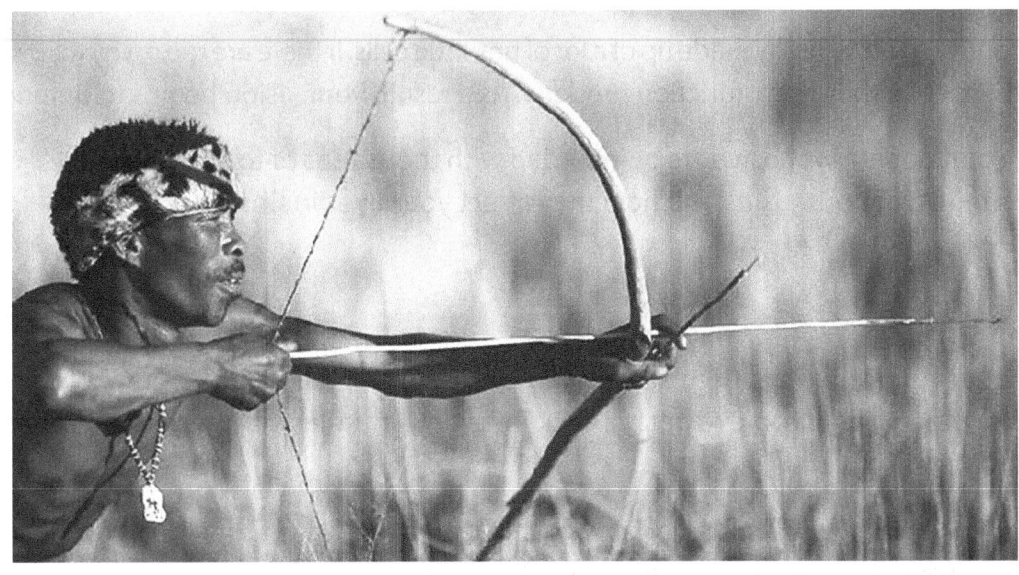

Research a couple years back showed that men tend to have better distance vision and women have better near vision. The researchers related the discrepancy to our respective roles in hunting and gathering. Men, the primary hunters, required the ability to see clearly across a vast field to bag the dinner. Women as primary foragers benefited from strong visual acuity up close as they located and then discerned edible from inedible plants.

If we study traditional hunter-gatherers, which are still found in remote regions of the earth, we find a surprising picture.

According to Dr. Loren Cordain, vision impairments are virtually nonexistent. Statistics in these traditional groups for myopia settle out at 0 to 3% and consist of almost exclusively mild cases.

If we look at statistics from modern societies, we find a much different picture. The numbers for myopia, for example, have skyrocketed in the last thirty years. In the U.S., the prevalence of myopia is 42%.

This virtually proves that genetics have little to nothing to do with poor vision. So what's the real cause?

Although there are many factors, here are the main 3:

1 Diet & Toxins

Although you might not hear it often enough, diet plays a significant role in the quality of your eyesight. In particularly, processed foods and other toxins.

Modern food isn't really food and doesn't nourish the eyes. Not only does this screw-up your eyesight, it also destroys your overall health.

Many of the toxins we are exposed to everyday, can impair our vision.

Your eyes are basically made up of a lot of tiny little cells. If there are too many toxins around these cells, they don't function properly. As a result, your vision begins to deteriorate.

In our modern world, we are bombarded with thousands of toxic chemicals. I'll go more into detail about toxins and how they affect your eyes in Chapter 6.

2 Eye Malnourishment

Your eyes need key nutrients to function properly. In fact, studies have shown nutrition plays a crucial role in eye health. Lack in key eye nutrients is the leading cause of eye problems.

Unfortunately, with industrial farming and commercialized food, you just aren't getting the nutrients your eyes require to function properly.

Later in the book I will show you the exact nutrients and amounts you need to supplement.

1   Bad Eye Habits

We just don't use our eyes the way we used to. In the past, we roamed outdoors and used both our short and long-range vision. Today, we spend almost all our time staring at a TV or a computer screen. As a result, millions of adults who should have healthy vision now have nearsightedness.

Smart phones seem to be the worst culprits. Researchers have identified a couple of reasons behind smart phone eyestrain. Because of the tiny screens and smaller fonts used on smart phones, the researchers found people generally hold their smart phones closer to their eyes than they would printed text.

What does this mean for us techno-suckers? Because of the size and distance, our eyes have a harder time focusing on the print. The strain involves two processes called accommodation – the adjustment from near to far distance; and vergence – eye movement toward and away from one another.

Modern lifestyles are especially setting up our children for strain as well as poor eye health. The diminished physical activity level and high screen time of many children's days have been connected with narrower blood vessels in the eyes, a characteristic of various common eye problems.

My point is, we just aren't using our eyes the way they're designed to be used. It's basically a matter of "Use-it or Lose-it".

When was the last time you went out for a walk and actually looked at the horizon line, looked pasted the numerous amounts of buildings and skyscrapers and actually used your long-range vision?

It's no wonder more and more people are getting diagnosed with these eye conditions.

These are the factors that determine the quality of your eyesight. Don't worry if it's all a little confusing at this point. What's important to understand is that poor vision has almost nothing to do with genetics.

The real reason your eyesight is poor is because of poor eating habits & toxins, malnourishment and just not using your eye muscles enough.

In the next part of this book, I'll show you the simple 3-Step solution to restore your perfect 20/20 vision.

PART 2
THE SOLUTION

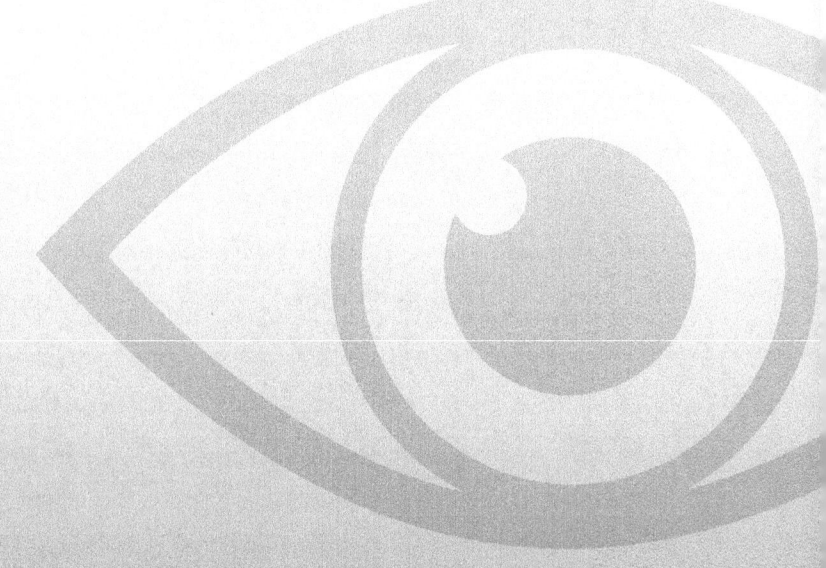

The Quantum Vision System is simple and easy to use. I worked really hard to make this accessible to as many people as possible. My goal is to end eye disease for good!

Here is a breakdown of the 3-Part System and how they work together to help you get the best eyesight you've ever had.

STEP 1

Optimize Your Diet & Cleanse

» Eat a nutrient rich diet the human body was designed for

» Cleanse your body and eyes from chemicals and pollutants

STEP 2

Nourish Your Eyes

» Add compounds that reverse & repair damaged eye cells

» Supplement key nutrients your eyes need for optimal sight

STEP 3

Eye Strengthening Exercises

» Follow the daily Quantum Vision Exercises to restore your vision naturally

» Have an eye condition? Cure it naturally with a specific eye exercise routine

It's time to learn the secret to natural eye restoration. Be sure to read the next few chapters carefully.

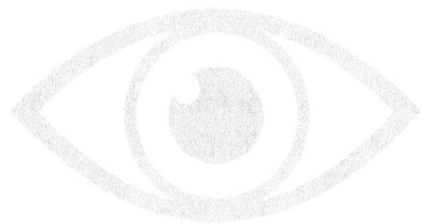

CHAPTER 5
OPTIMIZE YOUR DIET

Food for Vision

This is probably the most controversial section in the book. It flies in the face about everything we are taught in school about nutrition. It took me 15 years to discover what you're about to learn. And even though it's different from anything you've heard before, I can assure you that it's the TRUTH.

As you'll soon realize, our modern diet is so far from what humans were meant to eat. I'm surprised that there's not more sickness in the world. Thank God for our miraculous bodies which can deal with the punishment that we cause to ourselves through improper eating.

In this chapter I will show you what to eat to help to reverse your vision problems by giving your eyes the nutrients that they need.

Our Natural Diet

Many, many years ago, our ancestors lived a very different life. Although our digestive systems haven't evolved much since then, it is important to note that our diets have changed tremendously. In this section I will explain how these changes affect all of us.

There are basically two types of diets that humans thrive on. I'm going to share both with you. The first is by far the best diet for humans. It's just not an easy way to eat in our modern world. Luckily humans' second diet is easy to follow and gives you lots of choices. Remember, this is very different from what you have been taught in school, but stay with me. I promise it is worth it.

The Primary Human Diet

Many of us picture early man chasing animals and slaughtering them for food, then sitting around a campfire cooking meat with sticks. But is this true? Did ancient man eat a diet primarily of meat?

Before I answer that, look at what we learned in previous chapters about pharmaceutical companies. Remember, it's all about the profit. Is it possible that the pharmaceutical companies and big food companies and their lobbyists have affected the government food guidelines and what's taught in schools about food? You bet.

If you look at unbiased research and use logical thought, you'll quickly realize that thousands of years ago, people ate very little meat.

Let's imagine for a second that you've traveled back in time thousands of years and you're dropped in the middle of a field. How likely is it that you would catch an animal? Remember you don't have any fancy weapons.

Okay, let's say you have a spear and you're pretty good at using it. Well, even experienced hunters using old techniques have a very difficult time catching prey. On top of that you'd have to find something sharp to cut the meat and then build a fire.

Unless, of course, the thought of ripping open a little bunny with your bare hands and eating it to the bone with blood and other bodily fluids gushing all over you sounds enjoyable. An animal designed to eat meat wouldn't hesitate, so why should you? Because that would be wrong … right?

Let's do an experiment. Put a plate of raw meat and a plate of bananas in front of a young child or baby. Which one do you think it would eat based on pure instinct? Definitely the bananas.

It's my belief that if we were responsible for catching and killing animals for food, the majority of us would never eat meat again. The thought of killing another being is repulsive to most of us.

In fact, I think the evidence is very clear that humans were not primarily designed to eat meat.

You see, unlike animals that prey on and catch other animals for food, our teeth weren't designed to eat meat. Animals, such as tigers, have very sharp pointy teeth to rip through skin. We don't. Our teeth are basically flat – designed to chew or pulverize food.

The acid levels in meat eating animals are much higher than humans, which allow them to digest flesh. They can even manufacture their own vitamin C, something that humans need to get from the food they eat.

Also, animals that eat meat have very short digestive systems and even have stomachs designed for eating old meat that has been left out for days. Try doing that with a piece of uncooked chicken.

If you were to do a little research, you would find there are a vast number of differences between natural carnivores (meat eaters) and humans.

CHARACTERISTICS	HUMANS	CARNIVORES
Teeth	Short & Sharp	Flat & Spade Shaped
Chewing	Extensive Chewing Necessary	None, Swallows Food Whole
Tongue	Smooth	Rough
Legs	2	4
Nails	Flattened Nails	Sharp Claws
Sweat	Sweat From Pores	Sweat From Tongue Only
Stomach	Acidity With Food pH 4-5	Acidity With Food pH 1
Small Intestine	10-11x Body Length	3-6x Body Length
Colon	Long, Sacculated	Simple, Short & Smooth
Liver	Cannot Detoxify Vitamin A	Can Detoxify Vitamin A
Eating Habit	Repulsed By Raw, Old Meat	Loves Raw Meat, Even Days Old
Sleep	Sleep 33% Of Day	Sleep 80% Of Day
Vitamin C	Required From Food Sources	Makes Their Own Vitamin C
Arteries Clog	Yes, Low Tolerance For Fat	No, Thrive On High Fat

If we did eat meat, we ate very little of it. Usually it was scraps left over from other animals. But when we found it, we ate it all at once, since it's a high calorie food that goes bad. We'll get to why this is important later in the book.

In addition to not eating much meat, early man probably didn't consume any dairy products. Think about it, if you can't catch the cow, it's going to be very unlikely that you'll be able to drink its milk.

Did you know that humans are the only animals that consume milk after weaning? Moreover, humans do not drink human milk but drink the milk of other species … and do so throughout their adult lives. Does this seem natural to you?

What about grains? Do you think that early man ate wheat, rice, oats or rye? Humans can't chew or digest grains in their natural state. Grain-eaters (usually birds) have a pouch in their throats, where grains sit and germinate, thereby making them digestible. Humans cannot digest grains in their raw state.

What else is left? Vegetables, right? Yes, most likely.

However, they only ate raw vegetables, and since vegetables do not have many calories, there would not be enough substance in an all-vegetable diet.

Also, can you imagine a life of eating just vegetables all day? Especially with no dipping sauce or dressing? Talk about bland!

I know what you may be thinking. You need meat, dairy and grains to be healthy. My goodness … they're major food groups!

But wait … remember what we learned earlier. There's the real truth and then there is truth for profit. So what did early man eat? What did they naturally gravitate towards?

Before I get to that, let's talk about the qualities and characteristics of our ideal food.

Our ideal food would …

» Taste great raw and unseasoned
» Be easy to digest
» Be easy to find
» Nourish our body and supply it with enough vitamins and other nutrients required to live
» And have enough calories that our bodies crave and need

So what food satisfies all of the above?

There has been extensive research by scientists studying fossils of early man, specifically their teeth, to get an idea of what they ate and surprisingly this is what they found.

They ate a diet of almost entirely fruit!

When you research the preferences of animals that have the closest genetics to humans – the Bonobo chimpanzee – you will find too that their diet consists almost entirely of fruit.

While this might shock you, it does make sense and here's why:

1   Nutritionally, fruit comes closer to satisfying all of our needs than any other food.

2   Fruit tastes great raw, especially when it is ripe.

3   Fruit requires no preparation and is ready to eat in its natural state.

4   Fruit digests faster than any other food.

5   Fruit satisfies our desire for sweet tastes and smells.

6   When ripe, fruits convert carbohydrates into glucose and fructose – simple sugars that our bodies can use immediately without further digestion.

7   Fruits contain all the vitamins, minerals and enzymes that our bodies need to take energy from their sugar.

8   Fresh fruit is jam packed with Vitamin C. We are one of the only animals that don't manufacture our own Vitamin C. We have to get it from our diet in large quantities. (I'll talk about this later.)

9   Fruit is colorful and easy to find – just walk up to a tree and pluck it from a branch. In fact, once fruit is ready to eat, it falls to the ground. (No slaughtering necessary!)

10 Your brain is powered by, guess what, simple sugars. Fruit is the perfect food. There's even a lot of evidence to support our brains rapidly developed when we started eating fruit and since we've stopped, they've been slowly shrinking.

This may shock you, but by every indication, our digestive physiology was designed to process the soft, water-soluble fibers in fruits and tender leaves, also exclusively.

So what does this mean to you?

Does this mean that if you want to succeed with Quantum Vision System, you can no longer eat anything else but fruit?

Not at all. Luckily we are equipped with a secondary diet.

Our Secondary Diet

While it is true that a long, long time ago when we all lived near the equator we did eat almost entirely fruits. But many of thousands of years ago, humans did venture to colder climates and there, fruit was scarce.

In this point in evolution, fire and weapons were available, making catching prey much easier. Although still not optimal, our bodies started to evolve to digest meats and more vegetables.

As I mentioned earlier, humans can't manufacture our own Vitamin C. We have to eat foods with Vitamin C or we will die. You may have heard of a disease called scurvy that killed people who travelled by sea many years ago.

So what does the secondary human diet look like? Lots of meats, fish, healthy fats and vegetables. And some berries when available.

Although not ideal, it is much better than what most people eat today and a lot more sustainable.

REMEMBER TO CHOOSE HEALTHY MEATS

The way cattle is raised has changed tremendously in the last 50 years. Back then, animals were raised on small farms and ate the food God intended for them. Cows roamed large fields and ate their natural food – grass. They were healthy, strong and very lean on fat. Not only that, their fat was much different than it is today.

Grass fed cows have fat in a 3:1 ratio of omega-6 to 3. Today's commercial farmed cattle have a ratio of 20:1. Why is this important? Omega-6 fats are fats that coat your cells and create inflammation in your body and hurt your blood. But omega-3 fats are free flowing and clear the blood of its stickiness.

Plus, since commercially farmed animals are cooped up in a cage and eat unnatural food, they're all sick. So the farmers inject them with a constant stream of antibiotics. Not to mention the growth hormones they use to make them bigger and fatter, which is faster for profits. All of this leads to health problems. When you eat meat, pick grass-fed organic meats when possible.

Good meats can be expensive, so instead of buying them from the grocery store, find a local farmer and buy direct. You'll be surprised at how cheaply you can get high quality, healthy meat when you skip the middleman.

Why Raw Vegetables Are So Important?

It's very important that you get large amounts of fresh, raw vegetables in your diet every day and here's why.

Below are 2 pictures of live blood under a Darkfield Microscope. The blood on the left is healthy blood. The blood cells are separated and strong so they can get through narrow spaces and keep your eyes and body oxygenated. On the right you see unhealthy blood. It's all clumped together making it hard to pass through your capillaries in your eyes.

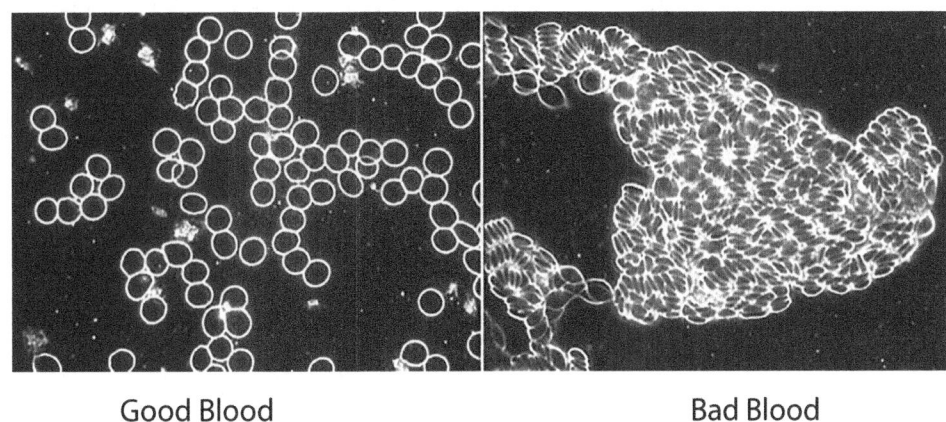

Good Blood   Bad Blood

But what causes your blood to stick together? Here I'll explain the importance of something called pH.

What we call pH is short for the potential of hydrogen. It is a measure of the acidity or alkalinity of our body's fluids and tissues. It is measured on a scale from 0 to 14. The more acidic a solution is, the lower its pH. The more alkaline, the higher the number is.

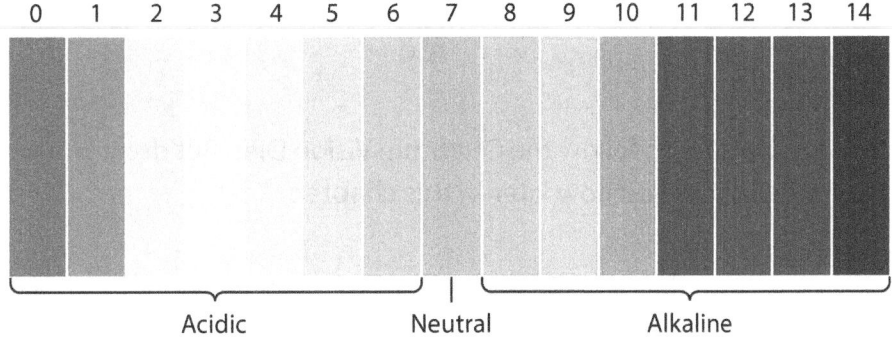

When your body is too acidic, your blood starts to clump together causing all sorts of problems including vision problems. The good thing is that it's easy to fix. You just need to adjust your diet to include more foods that are alkaline and fewer foods that are acidic. You can see where food fits into the pH scale in the diagram on the next page.

pH SPECTRUM

3	Carbonated Water, Club Soda, Energy Drinks	**7**	**Neutral pH** Most Tap Water, Most Spring Water, Sea Water, River Water
4	Popcorn, Cream Cheese, Buttermilk, Prunes, Pastries, Pasta, Cheese, Pork, Beer, Wine, Black Tea, Pickles, Chocolate, Roasted Nuts, Vinegar, Sweet and Low, Equal, Nutra Sweet	**8**	Apples, Almonds, Tomatoes, Grapefruit, Corn, Mushrooms, Turnip, Olive, Soybeans, Peaches, Bell Pepper, Radish, Pineapple, Cherries, Wild Rice, Apricot, Strawberries, Bananas
5	Most Purified Water, Distilled Water, Coffee, Sweetened Fruit Juice, Pistachios, Beef, White Bread, Peanuts, Nuts, Wheat,	**9**	Avocados, Green Tea, Lettuce, Celery, Peas, Sweet Potatoes, Egg Plant, Green Beans, Beets, Blueberries, Pears, Grapes, Kiwi, Melons, Tangerines, Figs, Dates, Mangoes, Papayas
6	Fruit Juices, Most Grains, Eggs, Fish, Tea, Cooked Beans, Cooked Spinach, Soy Milk, Coconut, Lima Beans, Plums, Brown Rice, Barley, Cocoa, Oats, Liver, Oyster, Salmon	**10**	Spinach, Broccoli, Artichoke, Brussel Sprouts, Cabbage, Cauliflower, Carrots, Cucumbers, Lemons, Limes, Seaweed, Asparagus, Kale, Radish, Collard Greens, Onion

This is why it's so important to follow the Quantum Vision Diet. But don't worry; it's easy and delicious to follow. I'll show you how later in this chapter.

Don't We Need Dairy For Our Bones?

Absolutely NOT. In fact, milk is one of the worst things that people can drink. The milk myth has spread around the world based on the flawed belief that this calcium-rich drink is essential to support good overall health and bone health. The confusion about milk's benefits stems from the fact that it contains calcium – around 300 mg per cup.

But many scientific studies have shown an assortment of detrimental health effects directly linked to milk consumption. And the most surprising link is that not only do we barely absorb the calcium in cow's milk (especially if pasteurized), but to make matters worse, it actually increases calcium loss from the bones. What an irony this is!

Knowing this, you'll understand why statistics show that countries with the lowest consumption of dairy products also have the lowest osteoporosis and fracture incidence rates.

But the sad truth is that most mainstream health practitioners ignore these proven facts. And they continue teaching children that you need milk for strong bones. Something the dairy industry has spent millions of dollars lobbying to congress.

While on the Quantum Vision System, I recommend that you stay away from dairy altogether. Instead, try unsweetened hemp milk, rice milk or almond milk. These great options are available at most supermarkets and health food stores.

What About Grains?

The same is true of grains. The problem with grains is that our bodies have difficulty digesting them. Our digestive systems weren't actually designed to eat them! In fact, we only started eating them about 10,000 years ago according to researchers. On top of that, the grains we eat today are far worse than what our ancestors ate. By the time we eat them, most grains have been ...

>> Stripped of most of their nutrients

>> Sprayed with toxic pesticides

>> Surrounded by fertilizer made primarily out of crude oil and since crops cannot utilize these synthetic minerals properly, much of our crops are nutrient deficient like the soil

>> Irradiated which kills any remaining life in them, essentially making them dead food

>> Some crops such as corn are grown from heavily genetically modified seeds, which have been linked to numerous health issues

And that's not all. Once they're harvested, instead of using stone mills as they used to, they use high-speed metal presses that grind everything into a fine powder. This flour causes our blood sugar to spike really quickly and actually depletes our body of nutrients. By the time grains have been through all this processing, they have up to 90% less nutrients.

The Quantum Vision Diet

The Quantum Vision Diet has been designed to reverse your poor vision. The following are guidelines, which you should follow. It's important to follow the diet, as we are trying to enrich your body with the nourishment it needs to get perfect 20/20 vision.

Breakfast

As we learned in the previous section, early humans ate mostly fruit. So it's important to eat some fruit each and every day. Remember, your body is designed to run on fruit.

The best time to eat fruit is in the morning for breakfast. You were essentially fasting during the night, and the best way to break a fast is at breakfast (That's where the word break-fast comes from).

You can eat any fruit you want and in any quantity. There are just 2 things to remember.

1   It's best to eat one fruit at a time. You don't have to, but it's easier for your body to digest. Ideally, if you want grapes one morning, eat only grapes. The next day, pick another fruit or the same fruit, just as long as you only eat one fruit at a time.

2   Try to eat ripe fruit. Eat bananas when they're spotted. Eat fruit when it's sweet and juicy. It can be hard to find good ripe fruit. Modern farming and shipping practices make everything taste like potatoes. Try smaller fruit markets, they tend to have the best fruit. Try to choose fruits that are in season and grow locally.

That's it. Just start each day with some fruit.

NOTE: This is the most healing diet. Period. I recommend 100% fruit diet (breakfast/lunch/dinner) if you are having severe health problems, as it is the FASTEST way to heal. If you find that you are not improving on the standard diet, do a fruit cleanse for 7 days. Nothing but fruit. Otherwise, continue with the fruit in the morning and mixed meals for the rest of the day.

Lunch/Dinner

Lunch and dinner are just as easy. Instead of fruit, we are going to switch to our secondary diet of meat and vegetables. Here are the rules, they're simple:

1   Vegetables should be raw (uncooked). The best way to do this is just eat a big salad with lunch and dinner.

1   Follow the 80/20 principle. 80% of your meal should be vegetables, and 20% high quality meat.

2   When buying meats, try to buy grass-fed, free-range meats that are hormone and anti-biotic free.

Foods To Avoid

Remember; avoid these foods at ALL times while on the Quantum Vision Diet because they contain foods that cause eye problems.

JUNK FOOD		
All Dairy	All Grains	All Desserts
All Fast Food	All Processed Sugar	All Toxic Additives
All Processed Food (breakfast cereals, bread, white rice, pasta, microwave meals, soft drinks, pizza, French fries, Granola bars, canned meat, hot dogs, lunch meat, store bought salad dressing etc.)		

That's it! It's that simple. Just eat fruit in the morning, and vegetables and healthy meat for lunch and dinner. If you want to accelerate your healing, just eat fruit only for the first week.

Following this simple meal plan will go a long way to improving your health and restoring your vision to a perfect 20/20!

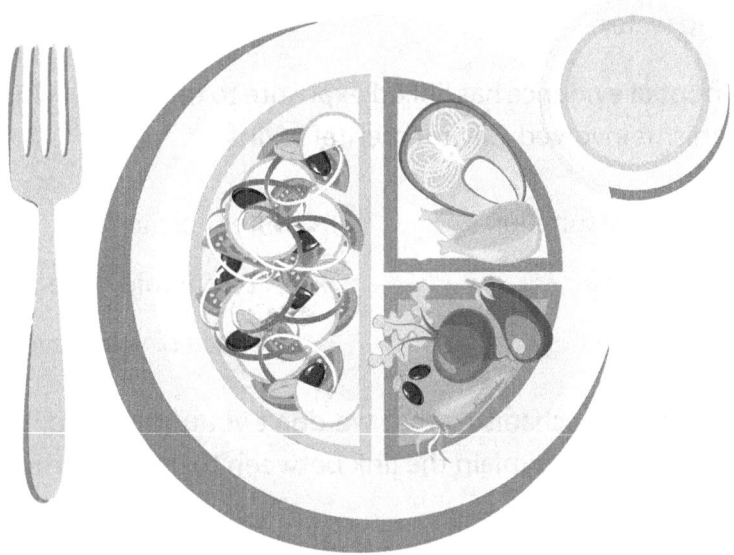

CHAPTER 6

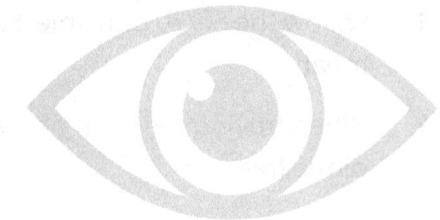

CLEANSE YOUR EYES

First Thing's First – Reduce Your Toxic Load

We don't tend to think of our environment as something that causes us to have health problems, but it does.

Environmental factors such as toxins contribute to vision problems. These toxins cause all sorts of health problems and they're in everything. In today's modern society, it's next to impossible to avoid all of them.

Toxins and Vision Problems

Each year, the toxic burden in our air, food and water (and therefore our bodies) grows higher and higher. Companies manufacture 6.5 trillion pounds of 9,000 different chemicals each year. And the same companies release over 7 billion pounds of 650+ different pollutants into the atmosphere and water.

An increasing amount of evidence has linked exposure to toxins with vision problems. There are several mechanisms involved. Environmental toxins:

>> Disrupt mitochondrial function

>> Cause oxidative stress

>> Promote inflammation

>> Alter hormones

>> Alter thyroid metabolism

>> Reduce oxygen levels

There are probably other mechanisms that we don't yet understand. But the ones I listed above are certainly enough to explain the link between toxins and vision problems.

The most obvious first step is to remove all food toxins from your diet. This means ditching processed and refined foods, industrial seed oils, high fructose corn syrup, as well as anything you can't pronounce.

The second step is to take steps to reduce your exposure to chemicals at home. This means choosing non-toxic household cleaners.

When you reduce your exposure to these chemicals and eat the Quantum Vision Diet, you'll restore your body's natural capacity to be Glasses Free!

Here's what to avoid:

1   Smoking

There are more than 600 ingredients in a cigarette. When burned, tobacco smoke contains more than 7000 chemicals. Many of these chemicals are poisonous and at least 69 of them are known to cause cancer[1].

Smoking actually damages the feedback mechanism in the liver that controls the amount of cholesterol made by the body[2], leading the body to create even more cholesterol. This can contribute to unhealthy blood.

Even if you don't smoke, you can be exposed to the chemicals in cigarette smoke. In fact, some chemicals in secondhand smoke have been found in even higher concentrations[3].

The best option is to quit smoking altogether and avoid secondhand smoke whenever possible. Your body and your family will thank you.

2   Toxic Food

Processed foods are loaded with additives, preservatives, artificial sweeteners, flavors and trans-fats that are toxic to your body.

Most meat that we buy at the grocery store is high in toxins as most farm animals eat toxic food that accumulates toxins in their bodies. Naturally raised and organic meat is less inflammatory to the body, as the animals are fed a more natural diet and have higher levels of anti-inflammatory omega-3 fatty acids.

Even fruits and vegetables can be covered in chemicals, such as hormone-disrupting pesticides. Choose fresh, organic produce, preferably from a local farmer.

Another major factor is not eating enough fruits and vegetables, the foods we were meant to eat. Eating too much meat, dairy and grains taxes the body and leads to inflammation.

Lastly, avoid anything that is GMO or Genetically Modified Food. Think about this, every study funded by the companies that produce GMO food say it's totally safe, but every study that is independently funded says that GMOs are extremely toxic. You decide. Whenever possible eat organic!

1   Refined Sugar

When they say sugar is everywhere, it's because it is. Sugar is one of the main ingredients in your fruit juices, soft drinks and sports drinks, and is even hidden in nearly every junk and convenience food, including luncheon meats and prepared sauces and condiments.

Refined sugar is like poison to your body. It increases inflammation and slows down the healing process. Not to mention that the calories in sugar are essentially "empty."

It's important to read food labels very carefully. If the label says glucose, sucrose, maltose, lactose, fructose, corn syrup or white grape juice concentrate, extra sugar has been added.

If you want something sweet, eat a piece of fruit. And get in the habit of using natural sweeteners, such as honey or maple syrup, instead of white or brown sugar.

2   Unhealthy Fats

Damaged fats are one of the most dangerous foods that we can eat.

And what's crazy is that many of the most dangerous fats are the ones that we've been told to eat to be healthy. We've been taught that all vegetable fats are good. But in fact, these are some of the most poisonous things that we can put into our bodies.

The worst types of fats are hydrogenated fats, which are made by forcing hydrogen gas into oil at a very high temperature. Examples of hydrogenated fats are margarine and shortening.

Avoid at all costs margarine (even if the label says it's made from olive oil), soybean oil, corn oil, safflower oil, canola oil, vegetable oils and any oil that has been heated to a high heat, any oil that is sold in a clear bottle.

Other less common sources of fats that you will need to avoid include bottled salad dressings, baked goods, ice cream, chocolate, candy and snack foods such as potato chips.

1   Alcohol

Heavy drinking increases your risk of poor vision, even three drinks can increase your risk.

Alcohol acts as a depressant to the nervous system. A few drinks will block messages between the brain and the rest of the body. Chronic use of alcohol can damage blood vessels and reduce blood flow throughout the body too.

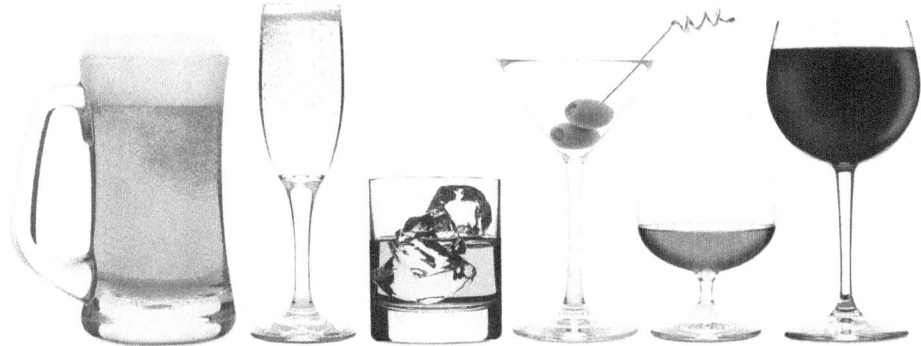

When at all possible, avoid consuming alcohol, or limit yourself to a couple of glasses per week.

2   Plastic

Most of us know by now to avoid toxic, plastic beverage bottles, plastic food storage ware, plastic wrap and resealable (or zipper lock) food storage bags. (If you didn't know that, now you do!) Plastic is everywhere, so you can't avoid it altogether. But you can limit your exposure.

Bisphenol A (BPA) and phthalates are dangerous chemicals that are used in the manufacturing of plastic products. Both have been shown to have an impact on hormones – basically by lowering testosterone.

It's a bit too much to get into in this book, but a quick search on Google will give you easy ways to reduce your plastic use.

3   Toxic Home and Personal Products

Personal Care Products: Have you ever really looked at the ingredients in your everyday lotion, soap or shampoo?

I bet you can't pronounce most of the ingredients in them. If you can barely understand what you are reading, imagine what these chemicals are doing to your body. Not to mention the warnings to not get the contents in your eyes! Everything that you put on your skin gets absorbed into your bloodstream and spreads throughout your body.

There are tons of all natural products out there, which contain readable ingredients that are good for you. From now on use only natural soap, detergent and moisturizer, etc.

And ladies, any eye makeup that you put on your eyes can end up IN your eyes. All the pigment, stabilizers and plastics, at some point or another, drop into eyes.

Natural cleaning supplies: Cleaning your house is a chore that needs to be done. But most of your cleaning supplies are full of harsh chemicals. These chemicals may make your kitchen or bathroom shine, while also killing bacteria, but at what cost to your health?

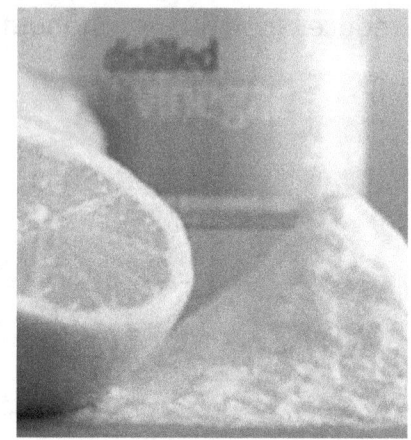

Did you know that unlike food, beverages and personal care products, cleaning products are not required by law to list their ingredients? Even if the chemicals in the bottles cause skin rash, asthma or even cancer, they don't need to tell you. Scary, right?!

So why not switch to all-natural cleaning supplies. The ingredients are usually well known and easy to pronounce such as; vinegar, lemon and baking soda.

1   Dirty Water

Tap water is loaded with chemicals. In addition to the chemicals that the city adds, such as chlorine and fluoride, most tap water contains prescription drug residue that the city can't clean out.

Got chlorine in your water? Most likely, since it's commonly used in municipal water treatment programs.

Chlorine is also in the hot spray of your morning shower, which means that you're absorbing it through your skin and eyes AND breathing it into your lungs. A quick fix is to buy a shower filter at your local hardware store. This will cost around $40.

Choose filtered water to drink. Drink lots throughout the day. In fact, most people are dehydrated and don't even know it. Here's how to find your ideal water intake: take your weight in pounds and divide it by 30. This is the number of ounces of water you should be drinking each day.

Weight (in pounds)	Divide by 30	= Number of 16-oz glass/day

1 Bad Air Quality

Let's face it. We can't control every molecule of air in our home. Regular dusting, sweeping and vacuuming can help. But the best and easiest way is to add more plants. NASA has been researching the power of common plants for years. Plants are particularly well suited for processing the benzene, formaldehyde and trichloroethylene in our indoor environments. Here are a few of the more common winners: English ivy, snake plants, spider plants, peace lily and golden pathos.

2 Pharmaceutical Drugs

If you are having problems with your vision, you may want to take a look at your medicine cabinet first. There are a number of prescription and over-the-counter drugs that may cause vision problems. These drugs definitely have a negative effect on your hormones, nerves, or blood circulation, resulting in less than perfect vision.

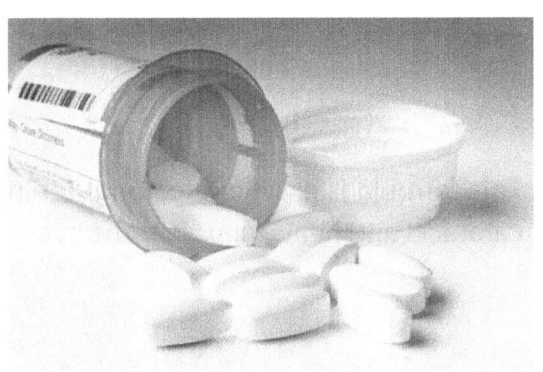

Talk to your doctor about getting off any prescription drugs (If possible).

3 Poor Sleep

Sleep is an incredibly regenerative time when your body repairs and detoxifies itself. If you're making the effort to reduce all the toxins in your environment but you're still not sleeping enough, you are losing out on the benefits.

Studies have shown that not getting enough sleep can have a huge impact on your hormones and stress levels. Everyone has different sleep needs. A general rule of thumb is to aim for 6-8 hours per night. Or, if you want to find out what your natural sleep requirements are, try going to sleep at the same time for two to three nights and wake up without an alarm clock. This will tell you roughly how much sleep you need each night.

This is by no means an extensive list. There are literally thousands of chemicals that you should avoid. And not just for your eyes but for your general health as well. If you want to get more information, I suggest you check out these books:

» Super Natural Home   » Toxin Toxout

» The Healthy Home   » Detoxify Or Die

Eye Cleansing (For Cataracts)

Now that you have a general idea to avoid toxic chemicals, we need to address the chemicals already trapped in your body and your eyes. I have discovered a powerful natural cleanse that will pull out toxins and impurities and sediments that are stuck in your eyes.

Doing this cleanse regularly will clean out your eyes and improve your vision by nourishing your optic nerves.

Just remember, it will cause a burning sensation. Unfortunately, it needs to be this powerful to remove toxic buildup that leads to conditions such as cataracts.

Eye Cleanse

This formula is excellent for brightening and healing the eyes, and it's known to remove cataracts and heavy film from the eyes.

What You'll Need

One Part Each:

» Bayberry Bark (⅛ tsp.)

» Eyebright Herb (⅛ tsp.)

» Golden Seal Root (⅛ tsp.)

» Red Raspberry Leaves (⅛ tsp.)

» Cayenne pepper (⅛ tsp.)

Instructions

1   Make this into a tea and put it into a glass eye cup. (Make sure it cools down.)

2   Tilt you head forward and place the filled cup on your eye.

3   While holding the cup in place, tilt your head back or lay down. NOTE: There will be a slight burning sensation when using the cayenne in the eye at first, but there is nothing to be concerned about.

4   Move your eye around gently to ensure the fluid gets to every part.

1   Do this 3-6 times per day for each eye.

2   Finally, drink ½ cup of the remaining tea, once in the morning and once at night. (Make extra tea, do not use tea you put in your eye.)

Notes

You may feel stinging during the wash. Your eyes may produce tears. This is your body's way of expelling toxins and residues. It is completely normal, so don't worry. Your eyes will sting less when they are closed.

After the treatment, you may experience some vision blurriness. This is why you should relax when the treatment is over!

IMPORTANT

DO NOT DO THE EYE CLEANSE IF YOU HAVE AN EYE INFECTION, HAVE HAD RECENT SURGERY ON THE EYES OR ANY LASER VISION CORRECTION OR ARE USING MEDICATIONS FOR YOUR EYES.

CHAPTER 7

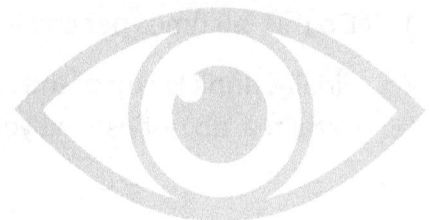

NOURISH YOUR EYES

Specific Nutrients for Your Eyes

As you learned in the previous chapters, eating a natural diet and reducing toxins is key to restoring your vision. But with industrial farming and the commercialization of food, it's next to impossible to get all the nutrients you need for perfect vision.

Unfortunately, if you already have poor vision, your eyes have been malnurished for quite some time.

In order to rebuild your eyes and restore perfect vision, we are going to need the help of some powerful herbs and essential vitamins and minerals. For many people, restoring eyesight just isn't possible without these supplements.

I can't stress how important these ingredients are to the program. Without them, I can't guarantee your success with the Quantum Vision System.

We've had thousands of people go through the program and I can guarantee you these ingredients are powerful, and the results for eyesight are nothing short of extraordinary.

Let's look at the individual ingredients to understand their true potential.

Ingredients

1. **Beta Carotene** – Beta carotene is important because it converts into Vitamin A, which helps against all sorts of eye diseases. Vitamin A protects your eyes and allows them to function properly and efficiently. A lack of vitamin A can lead to night blindness, near-sightedness, and even glaucoma.

2. **Vitamin C** – Vitamin C is considered an important vitamin because it is an antioxidant. Antioxidants help protect cells against damage from aging, which is important for preventing Cataracts, Macular Degeneration and corneal ulcers.

3. **Vitamin E** – Vitamin E works with Vitamin C to keep healthy tissues strong. Vitamin E can help fight against Cataracts and Macular Degeneration, and in some cases has been shown to stop the disease from developing further.

4. **Copper** – Copper has been studied as a nutrient to improve eye health. Specifically, copper has been used to help reduce the development of advanced age-related Macular Degeneration and now many ophthalmologists recommend it.

5. **Zinc** – Zinc is an important mineral as it helps keep the retina of your eye in working condition. Zinc is a hard mineral to get, and most people lack zinc in their diet.

6. **Lutein** – Lutein helps protect against eye damage, by absorbing into the lens and retina of your eye. They help fight against damage from sunlight, cigarette smoke and air pollution, while reducing your risk of Macular Degeneration and Cataracts.

7. **Zeaxanthin** – Zeaxanthin is a powerful, natural antioxidant that protects the eye from absorbing damaging blue light and reducing glare. Blue light can cause harmful oxidative stress in the eye. Zeaxanthin protects cells and membranes by reducing harmful free radicals.

8. **Bilberry** – Bilberry helps reverse retinopathy (damage to the retina) because anthocyanosides appear to help protect the retina. Bilberry has also exhibited protective effects against Macular Degeneration, Glaucoma, and Cataracts.

9. **Bayberry Bark** – Bayberry bark reduces inflammation in and around the eyes. It also reduces pain and secretion of excess fluids.

10. **Golden Seal Root** – Golden seal root helps reduce eye irritation and prevent eye infections.

11. **Red Raspberry Leaf** – Red raspberry leaf contain anthocyanins that help you see in dim light. They also protect eye tissue from oxidative or stress-induced cell death.

12. **Marshmallow Root** – Marshmallow root as soothing, softening and calming properties. It reduces inflammation and swelling.

13 **Eyebright Extract** – Eyebright extract has a long history of use for eye problems, hence the name of Eyebright. When used appropriately, eyebright will reduce inflammation in the eye caused by blepharitis (inflammation of the eyelash follicles) and conjunctivitis (inflammation or infection of the membrane lining the eyelids).

14 **Cayenne Pepper** – Cayenne pepper improves blood circulation to get all of these ingredients to your eye tissues.

All of these **come together to form the Quantum Vision Miracle Mix.**

How These Supplements Work

This vision miracle mix is based on over three decades of research and combines these discoveries into a powerful, vision supplement.

It works synergistically at three levels to drastically improve your eyesight and heal the underlying problem that caused your poor vision in the first place. Simply put, this is how it works:

1 **Reduce Inflammation**

First, for instant results, Bayberry Bark, Marshmallow Root, and Eyebright work together to reduce inflammation in and around the eye. This is what makes this supplement work so effectively and so quickly.

2 **Remove Toxins**

Next, Bilberry, Goldenseal Root, Red Raspberry Leaf and Cayenne Pepper work together to clear out any existing toxins within your eyes that are blocking nutrients. This can take some time depending on how toxic your eyes are. That's why we recommend taking this supplement for at least 3 months.

3 **Supply Nutrients**

Finally, high dose Vitamins, Minerals, Lutein and Zeaxanthin nourish the cells in your eyes so they regrow to strengthen your vision. Again it can take some time for your body to repair the damage caused from years of deficiencies, so take the supplement for at least 3 months. Ideally, you would continue taking the supplements for a year or more to clear out all the toxins and protect yourself from age related vision loss.

How To Make The Quantum Vision Shake

I've tried to make this as simple as possible, but you need all these ingredients to make the formula work. You can find these ingredients for purchase on the Internet, or even at your local health food store.

Make sure all ingredients are either organic or wildcrafted. It's important all these ingredients are of the highest quality or they may not be effective:

Ingredients

- Beta Carotene (10 mg)
- Vitamin C (400 mg)
- Vitamin E (70 mg)
- Copper (5 mg)
- Zinc (15 mg)
- Lutein (10 mg)
- Zeaxanthin (10 mg)

- Bilberry (50 mg)
- Bayberry Bark (50 mg)
- Golden Seal Root (35 mg)
- Red Raspberry Leaf (20 mg)
- Marshmellow Root (20 mg)
- Eyebright Extract (85 mg)
- Cayenne Pepper (20 mg)

Directions

Add all ingredients into a 8oz glass of your favorite juice or water and mix with a spoon. Drink immediately.

Take the Miracle Mix 2x per day. Once before breakfast and once before dinner. The best time to take it is **30 minutes before a meal.**

Ideally, you should continue taking these supplements everyday, even after your eye problems improve or are eliminated. That way you will continue to have perfect 20/20 vision.

Supplier Disclaimer

Before making the mix, please research all ingredient brands and suppliers. Unfortunately, we cannot guarantee the effectiveness of Quantum Vision when using ingredients souced from unknown suppliers for the following reasons:

1. You cannot be certain of the safety of the ingredients (many suppliers use ingredients contaminated by pecticides and other toxic chemicals).

2. You cannot be certain about the quality or potency of these products because they may or may not have been tested for strength and effectiveness.

3. You cannot be certain the ingredients have not been damaged due to high speed manufacturing practices. (High heat destroys these ingredients).

How Much Do You Need?

This is a tough question since I don't know your medical history, how long you've had trouble with your vision, or how closely you'll stick to the recommended diets. Having said that, I've put together some guidelines based on what I've learned while working with former customers who have gone through the program.

CURRENT VISION	RECOMMENDED USAGE
Vision Issues Less Then 3 Years	3 Months
Vision Issues 3-7 Years	3-6 Months
Vision Issues For More Than 7 Years	6-12 Months

If you have any reservations about the ingredient suppliers or making the drink yourself, then we recommend you use SignGain. This is a supplement we produce that contains all of of the ingredients listed above at the highest quality and potency.

Why We Created SightGain

When we first started sharing The Quantum Vision System, we used to recommend specific third-party ingredient suppliers to help support the amazing results of the program. Unfortunately, over time, we began to recieve customer feedback on the effectiveness of the system.

Upon research, we discovered the quality of the ingredients from these suppliers was very inconsistent (due to lower quality ingredients to increase profits) and this lead to customers not seeing the results they expected.

This did not sit well with us.

Our corporate mission is to bring health and wellness alternatives to the masses - a revolutionary Vision System with products that ACTUALLY work, are of the highest quality and at a price point that consumers can afford. Naturally, we couldn't continue to recommend a substandard product to our customers.

Without any good alternatives, we decided to take matter into our own hands. We spent countless months sourcing the highest quality ingredients available and made sure our supplements were manufactured to the highest standards possible.

Research

All of these ingredients have been clinically tested and proven effective in double blind studies. They are the result of decades of research from leading universities and research firms around the world.

This is the real deal. It's been thoroughly tested for safety and effectiveness in thousands upon thousands of patients.

This stuff works. In fact, when combined, most of our customers see drastic improvements in their vision within 3 months of use.

If you're the type of person who likes to dig into research, you can view the papers and studies that lead to the discovery of the Quantum Vision System that are listed in the reference section at the end of this book.

After almost a year of our own internal research and testing, we created SightGain.

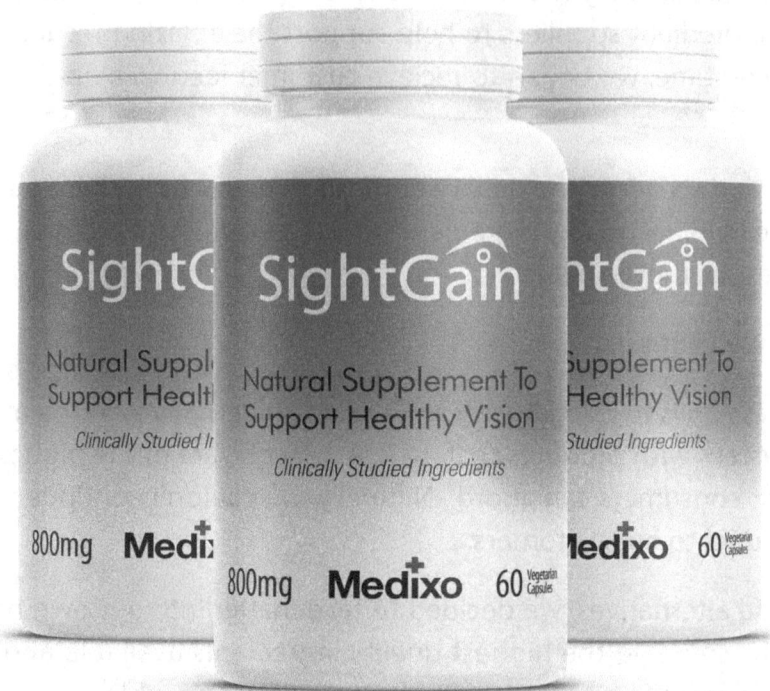

Not only does SightGain contain all the ingredients needed at effective dosages, it's also the most cost effective formula.

SigntGain is a product that we proudly and confidently stand behind. It contains the highest quality ingredients and has the strongest potency, so our customers can get the results we promise.

SightGain is the only guaranteed way to get all the specific herbs used for the mix at effective dosages. And it's available exclusively for Quantum Vision customers.

SightGain Directions:

Follow the directions specified on the bottle.

How To Get It

If you did not order a bottle of SightGain with your purchase of The Quantum Vision System, you can still get it.

FOR A LIMITED TIME: New customers are eligible for a 30% discount if you order within 7 days of purchasing The Quantum Vision System.

Note: It's made in small batches to ensure potency and quality, so sometimes they run out of stock. It's best to order as soon as possible, so you aren't delayed starting the Quantum Vision System. You can place your order on the site below:

www.GetSightGain.com/Discount

CHAPTER 8

BREAKING BAD EYE HABITS

We all have a bad habit we need to break. But did you know that you have bad eye habits too?

These bad eye habits could have created the eye condition that you have right now. Or you currently could be creating one as we speak. Below is a list of bad eye habits you should stop as soon as possible.

9 Bad Eye Habits You Need to Break

1. Rubbing Your Eyes

Did you know the skin around your eyes is one of the most sensitive skin areas on your body?

Rubbing your eyes can break tiny blood vessels under the skin's surface, which can cause puffy eyes, dark circles or droopy eyelids.

Not to mention rubbing your eyes, can also cause pressure to build up in your eyes, which can lead to all sorts of eye conditions.

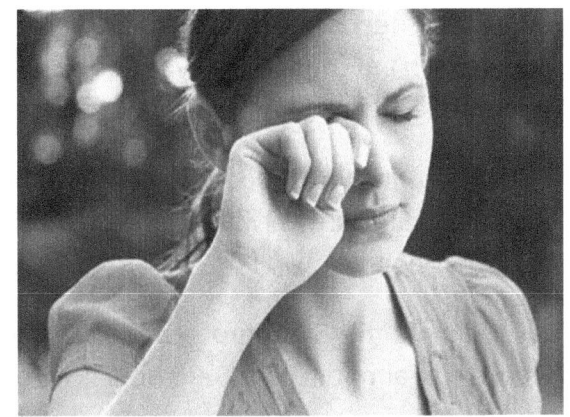

If you feel your eyes are becoming tired and you need to rub them, gently tap on the skin all around your eyes with your pointer and middle finger.

2. Wearing Sunglasses

We've all heard people nag about putting on sunglasses so the sun's UV rays won't damage your eyes, but the truth is, the sun is actually good for your eyes.

Avoid sunglasses when you're outdoors. Your eyes strengthen by adjusting to the changing light levels. Plus, you'll absorb more vitamin D. Just remember, the sun heals your eyes so get outdoors as much as possible.

Note: Although looking directly at the mid-day sun might be a no-no, looking at the sun during sunrise or sunset is the perfect way to stimulate your eyes.

3. Not Drinking Enough Water

Are you drinking the recommended 8 glasses of water a day? It may seem like a lot, but it's really necessary. Not drinking enough water and having a high-sodium diet can cause your body to dehydrate.

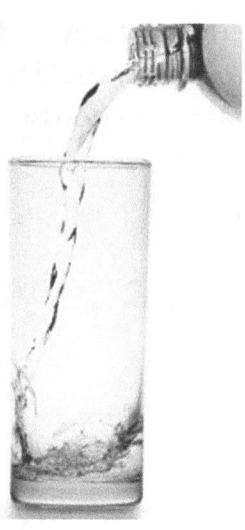

Your body (including your eyes) is made up of 70% water. If you become dehydrated, you are draining your eyes out of the moisture they need to create enough tears to stay healthy.

Symptoms associated with dehydration in the eyes are redness, puffy eyelids and dryness. If you find it hard to get enough water throughout the day, try setting an hour timer at your desk, when the timer goes off, finish your water glass and refill it. Add slices of Vitamin C-rich lemon or orange for a tasty boost.

4. Sleeping Poorly

Your body needs sleep to recoup after a hard day's work. Staying up late and getting up early doesn't allow the time your body needs to get into a deep realm of sleep, causing you to become achy and tired throughout the day.

But it's not just your body that shows you're lacking sleep, your eyes are usually the first sign. Dark circles, eye twitching, blurry vision, dry and red eyes are signs you are not getting enough sleep.

Try to aim for 6 – 8 hours of sleep each night. It's best to make this a routine, so even on the weekends, aim for those 6 – 8 hours!

The best part is your eyes are often the first to show you've had a good night sleep, giving you alert, glowing, bright eyes. So go get a good night's sleep tonight and reap the benefits tomorrow!

5. Not Giving Your Eyes Time To Breathe

If you have astigmatism, are nearsighted or far-sighted and wear glasses or contact lenses daily, give your eyes time to breathe. Don't wear your glasses all the time, take them off and do tasks that don't require them, such as reading a book if you are farsighted.

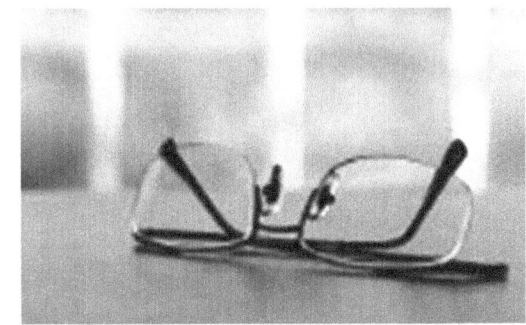

As we mentioned earlier in this book, most people get comfortable wearing their glasses all the time. This causes your vision to get worse. Seeing through a prescription made for farsightedness, to read a book up close, causes unnecessary strain to your eyes and deteriorates your vision. This is even more important with contact lenses, although they may be convenient; they are sitting directly on your eye.

Your eye needs oxygen to fight infection. If you wear contacts daily, you are at a greater risk of developing an eye infection or dry eyes, which can cause you to scratch your cornea due to the lens drying out. Always alternate between glasses and contacts, and take a break from both to really see the world from your own eyes.

6. Lying Down While Watching TV

When you watch movies or TV, do you lie down on the couch? It may not seem like something that hurts your eyes, but lying down while watching TV, puts serious strain on your eyes.

Your eyes aren't level with the TV; they are viewing the TV at an angle, which causes your eyes to try to focus on the image while flipping it right side up.

All the added strain is causing your vision to deteriorate. From now on, sit up on the couch while watching TV and while you are at it, sit at a good distance away from the TV screen.

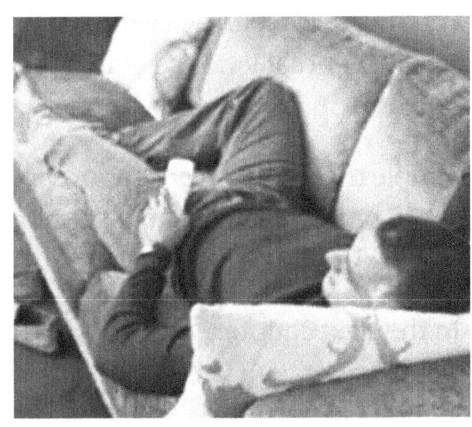

7. Reading in Poor Light

Everyone likes a good book in bed from time to time. But if you are reading in poor lighting you are hurting your eyes. Dim light while reading can make it difficult for your eyes to focus, causing short-term eye fatigue, dry eyes and blurred vision.

Always have a reading lamp on while reading. Invest in a low watt reading light for your bedside table, that way you can enjoy your book in bed, while not disturbing your partner.

8. Reading While Travelling

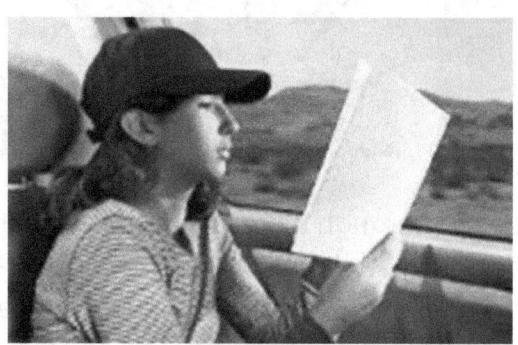

One of the worst things you can do for your eyes is reading while in a moving vehicle. It may get boring sitting on that train or during a road trip, but it puts strain on your eyes.

The unstable movement of the vehicle causes your eyes to keep adjusting. This can cause headaches, blurred vision, red and dry eyes. Next road trip try playing a car game with your friends!

9. Using Your Laptop to Watch Movies

We all know about the latest trend of watching movies or videos on your laptop or tablets, but did you know that these devices are causing your eyes to deteriorate? Since you are watching the screen at such a close distance from your eyes, you are putting unnecessary strain on your eyes, and causing them to focus on a bright screen from inches away.

In general, staring at any computer screen for too long can cause headaches, eye fatigue, eye dryness and red eye. If you find it hard to get away from your computer, tablet or smartphone, try the 20-20-20 trick. Every 20 minutes, look 20 feet away from your screen for 20 seconds. You'll eventually notice your eyes feel less tired and strained during the day!

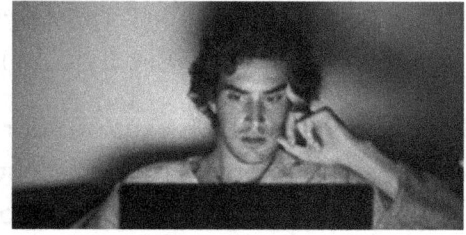

Simple tricks like the ones above can help you to break these bad eye habits and give your eyes the attention they deserve.

In the next chapter, we'll go into the simple eye exercises you can do throughout the day to help restore your vision and eliminate the workday strain from your eyes.

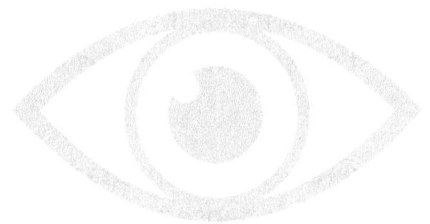

CHAPTER 9

QUANTUM VISION EYE EXERCISES

In this chapter I will show you how to perform each eye exercise step-by-step. In the next chapter I will show you how to stack them into routines for your specific eye condition.

I focused on the eye exercises that will help restore your vision. These techniques act like a workout for your eyes, strengthening your eye naturally.

Each exercise is useful in helping relieve eye stress or strain and help stimulate the flow of nutrients in the eye. Some of the exercises focus on improving your vision through sharpening your eyes ability to see detail, while others work on improving the control of your eye's extraocular muscles.

The exercises don't need a lot of time, and can easily be done throughout the day, without interrupting your daily activities.

IMPORTANT

DO NOT do these exercises without taking the supplements recommended in pervious chapters. The Quantum Vision eye exercises are designed to strengthen the muscles in your eyes, but without the supplements, your eyes won't heal fast enough to improve your vision and you won't get the breakthrough results you're expecting.

Note: Make sure to remove your glasses or contact lenses during exercises. If you want to work on maintaining a lower prescription, then wear your lowest prescription eyeglasses or contact lenses during the exercises.

If you follow the Quantum Vision System and really do the exercises, you can gradually improve any common vision problem, regardless of your age or circumstance.

So let's get started!

Pumping

Pumping is used to increase the flow of nutrients while exercising the focusing mechanisms of the eye.

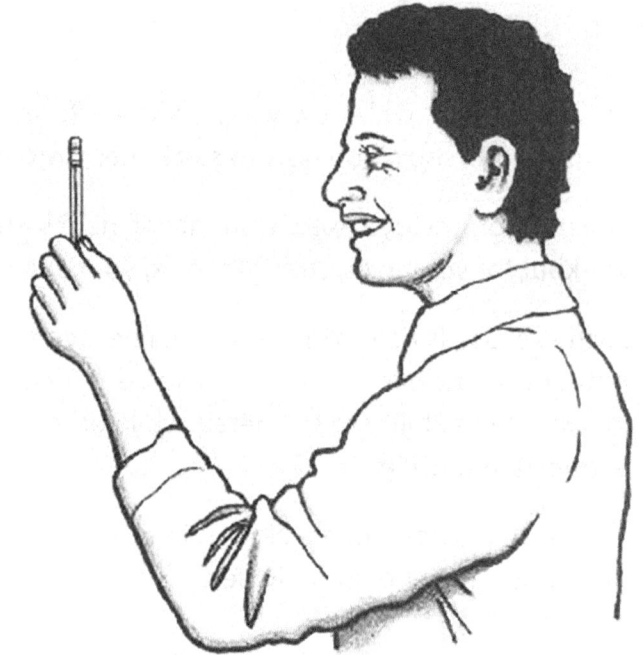

Directions

Hold an object 6 inches away from your face. This object can be your finger, a pen or another small object. *Change focus every two seconds* between the near object (finger or pen) and a far object at least 15 feet away, such as a tree, billboard, traffic lights, etc. Keep changing your focus back and forth between the near object and the far object.

Example

Pen – tree – pen – billboard – pen – truck – pen – traffic light.

Make sure to focus on a new far object each time.

Also make sure your near object is 6 inches away and no farther. Use a ruler to measure the distance of your near object if needed.

Try to briefly focus on a specific detail on both the near and far object before switching.

This exercise can easily be done during TV commercial breaks or office breaks.

If preforming this exercise indoors, you may use an object across the room. Such as a lamp, bookshelf corner or doorframe edge.

Tromboning

Like Pumping, Tromboning is also used to exercise the focusing mechanisms of the eye and increase the flow of nutrients.

Directions

Hold an object at arm's length away from your face. This object can be a finger or pen. ***Breathing slowly and deeply, look at the object*** as you move the object close towards your nose and then stretch your arm back out.

As you inhale, slowly bring the object in towards your face until it touches your nose – make sure to focus on the object. As you exhale, slowly take the object out to arm's length.

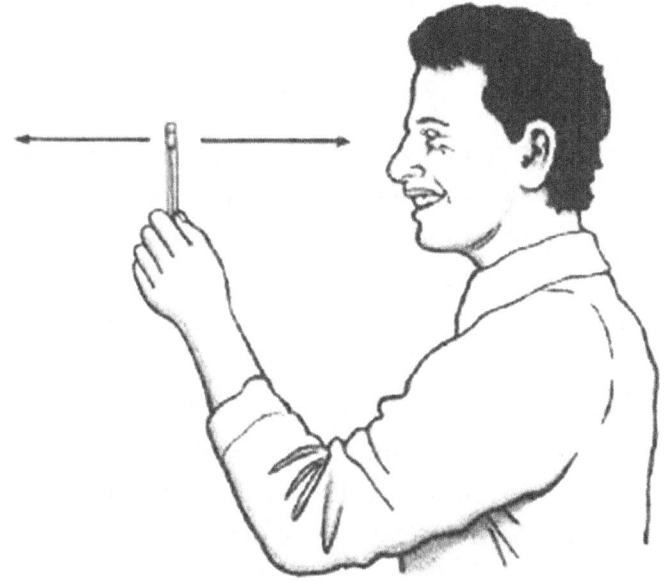

Example

Inhale – in towards nose, exhale – away from nose.

Make sure to time the movements with your breathing. It's important to have slow, deep breaths, so you aren't moving the object too fast.

When you bring the object close to your nose, you may notice the object going out of focus or forming a double image. Try to keep the object from going out of focus. Once you notice it happening, slow down the object and let your eyes focus on a small detail.

Continue the exercise for as long as possible, keeping the object in full focus the whole time.

Clock Rotations

Clock Rotations stimulate the flow of nutrients and help control the extraocular muscles around the eye.

Directions

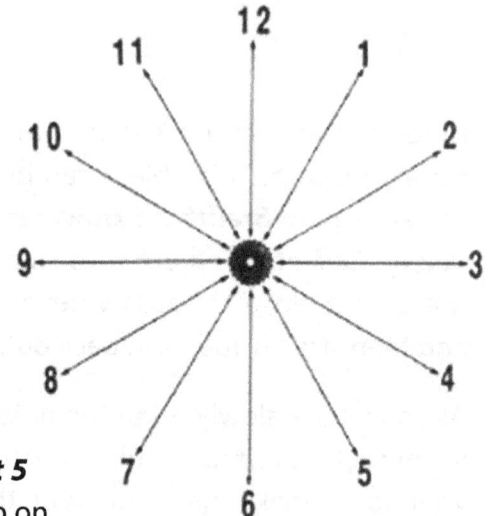

Hold an object comfortably at arm's length away from your face. Again this object can be a finger or pen. Now imagine that the object is in the center of a clock. 12 o'clock would be directly above it and 3 o'clock would be directly to the right of the object. Keeping your shoulders and neck still, look at the object, and extend your arm all the way up to 12 o'clock. ***Keep looking at the object for 2 -3 seconds. Then return to the center, and repeat this movement 5 times.*** Then move on to 1 o'clock, then 2 o'clock and so on.

Example

Up to 12 o'clock – hold for 3 seconds, repeat x5, up and slightly over to 1 o'clock – hold for 3 seconds, repeat x5, up and slightly over to 2 o'clock – hold for 3 seconds, repeat x5, to the right to 3 o'clock – hold for 3 seconds, repeat x5, etc.

Make sure to stretch the extraocular muscles as far as it will go in each clock position, before moving on to the next position.

It's important to keep the extraocular muscles fully stretched for the full 2- 3 seconds. If you notice a specific clock position that feels strained, repeat this specific position for another 5 times. Eventually it will become less strained.

Take your time, and slowly move around the clock. Do not rush this exercise. If you stretch the extraocular muscles too hard you will see flashes of light, this means you are stressing the retina.

Eye Rolls

Like Clock Rotations, Eye Rolls also stimulate the flow of nutrients and help control the extra-ocular muscles around the eye.

Directions

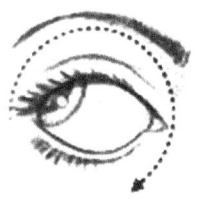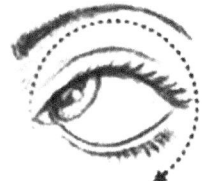

Slowly roll your eyes in a complete circle. First clockwise then, counterclockwise. Try to keep the extraocular muscles fully stretched throughout the entire rotation.

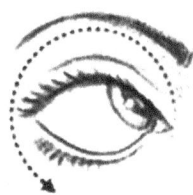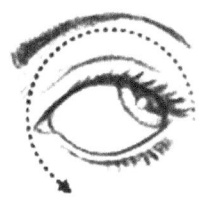

Don't look at anything in particular and slowly roll your eyes. We are working on coordination and control, without any jerkiness. If you feel strain or stress in a certain location, continue with the eye rolls until it becomes smoother.

Example

Eye roll clockwise, eye roll counterclockwise, eye roll clockwise, eye roll counterclockwise, etc.

Take your time, and slowly roll your eyes. Do not rush this exercise. If you stretch the extra-ocular muscles too hard you will see flashes of light, this means you are stressing the retina.

If you are easily motion sick, you may find yourself feeling unwell. Stop, cover your eyes with your hands, and continue the exercise with your eye opens.

Slow Blinking

Slow Blinking is used to reduce visual stress or strain.

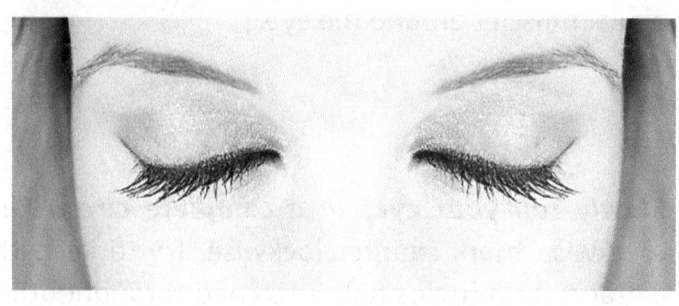

Directions

Start by breathing deeply and slowly. Once you feel comfortable and relaxed, do a few normal blinks when you inhale for the first time. As you exhale, close your eyes lightly. Exhale slowly allowing your eyes time to rest. When you inhale from now on, keep your eyes open. ***Close your eyes only on exhaling – creating a slow blink.***

Example

Inhale – open eyes, exhale – close eyes, inhale – open eyes, exhale – close eyes, etc.

When you inhale try to completely fill your lungs. When you exhale, slowly push all the air out of your lungs. Repeat this exercise until you feel free of all stress and strain on your body and eyes.

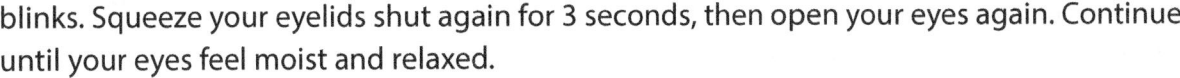

Squeeze Blinking

Squeeze Blinking is used to stimulate the production of tear fluid.

Directions

Squeeze your eyelids closed tightly for 3 seconds. Open your eyes wide and do a few normal blinks. Squeeze your eyelids shut again for 3 seconds, then open your eyes again. Continue until your eyes feel moist and relaxed.

Example

Squeeze close (hold 3 seconds), open, squeeze close (hold 3 seconds), open, squeeze close (hold 3 seconds), open, etc.

After a couple Squeeze Blinks your eyes will start to create an excess of tear fluid.

Try to isolate your eye muscles when you Squeeze Blink, and not scrunch or wrinkle your forehead or eyebrows.

Blur Zoning

Blur Zoning improves the eye's ability to see small details.

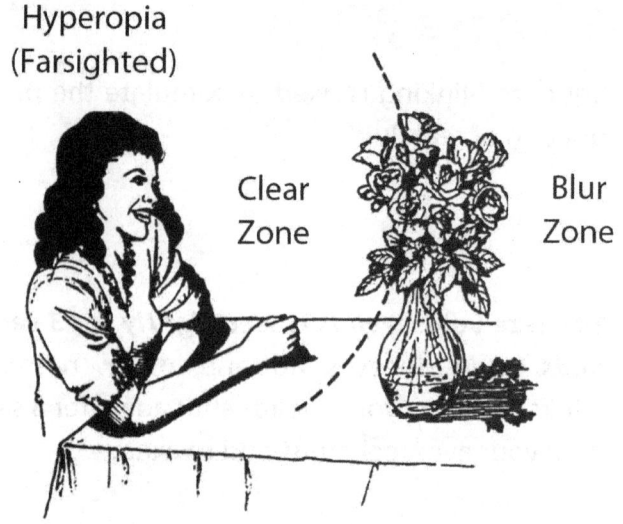

Hyperopia (Farsighted)

Clear Zone

Blur Zone

Directions

Find your Blur Zone in your vision – the spot where you can no longer see an image clear and crisp. Once you have found your Blur Zone, **focus your eyes around the edge of an object, following the major outlines.** Your object can be a tree in the distance if you are nearsighted, or a piece of jewelry held up close if you are farsighted.

Go slowly around the object 3 times. Then go around the object again, but this time really study the small details of the object and try to see the exact shape. Do this a couple more times around the object. Then go around the object again 3 times, this time really focusing on the smallest details on the object. If you are nearsighted and are looking at a tree, try to visualize a leaf while looking at a cluster of leaves. If you are farsighted, study a scratch, or metal imperfection on a piece of jewelry. Once you are finished the 3rd time around, rest your eyes.

Example

Follow the edge of an object – x3, follow the edge of an object – looking for details x3, then follow the edge of an object – looking for smaller details x3, rest your eyes.

While focusing around the edges of the object, follow the turns and cutouts the outline of the object makes.

Try not to squint to see any of the details. Just stay calm and relaxed and try to visualize smaller and smaller details on the object.

Shifting

Shifting is your eye's natural way of viewing objects. Like Blur Zoning, Shifting improves the eye's ability to see small details.

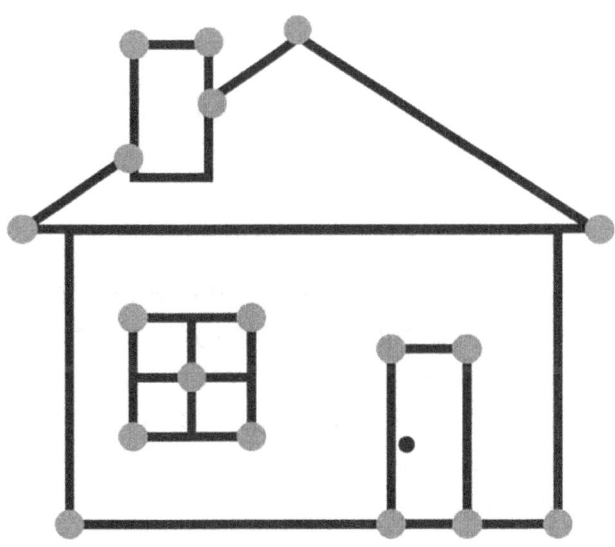

Directions

Using the image above as a guideline, focus your eyes on one dot. Now shift or move your focus from that one dot to the next closest dot. Continue doing this until every dot has been shifted to. Then start shifting from one random dot to another random dot on the image. From one corner to the other corner, the middle to the edge, etc.

Now use this method and focus on a real life object, like a house across the street, or bookcase. Don't imagine dots, but focus on specific areas of the object. First start by **shifting from one spot to a closer spot on the object**, then shift from a random spot to another random spot. Do this 3 times on 3 different objects. Once you are finished, make sure to rest your eyes.

Example

Shift from spot to close spot, shift from spot to close spot, shift from spot to random spot, shift from spot to random spot – x3, repeat on 3 different objects, rest your eyes.

Palming

Palming is used to relax your eye muscles and reduce visual stress or strain.

Directions

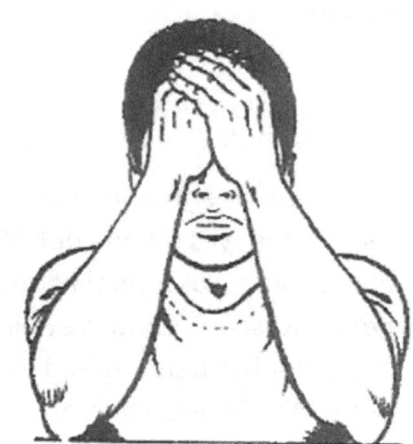

Close your eyes and place your left hand over your left eye, and your right hand over your right eye. You may lay your right fingers on top of your left fingers over your forehead. Rest the heel of your palms on your cheekbones and your elbows on a table. Rest your eyes and relax. Slowly breathing in and out for 30 seconds.

You may want to put a pillow under your elbows for comfort. Don't press on your eyes, eyelids, or eyebrows. Try to relax all your eye muscles.

Hydrotherapy

Like Palming, Hydrotherapy is also used to relax your eye muscles and reduce visual stress or strain.

Directions

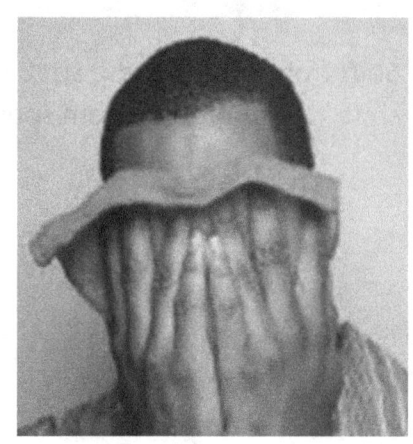

Grab three washcloths and two bowls. Fill one bowl with cold water, and fill the other bowl with hot water. Make sure the hot water is hot, but not scalding hot. The cold water should be ice cold. Now dip a washcloth in the hot water, close your eyes and ***hold the hot water washcloth against your eyes for 30 seconds.*** Now dip another washcloth in the cold water, close your eyes and ***hold the cold water washcloth against your eyes for another 30 seconds***. Continue switching between hot and cold washcloths every 30 seconds for 3 - 5 mins. Once you are finished gently massage your closed eyes with the dry washcloth.

Example

Hot washcloth – 30 seconds, cold washcloth – 30 seconds, hot washcloth – 30 seconds, cold washcloth – 30 seconds, etc. repeat for 3 - 5 mins, then massage with dry washcloth. Make sure to rest your eye muscles and don't push too hard on your eyelids.

Acupressure

Like Palming and Hydrotherapy, Acupressure is also used to relax your eye muscles and reduce visual stress or strain.

Upper Eye Socket

Close your eyes, place your thumbs on the inside of your upper eye socket, close to your nose, just below your eyebrow. The specific place usually feels like a boney ridge or nub. Once you have found the acupressure location, press firmly with your thumbs for one second, and then release for one second and repeat. Continue this for 30 seconds.

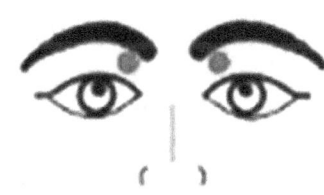

Example: press, release, press, release, press, release etc.

Bottom Eye Socket

Close your eyes and place your index and middle fingertips on the bottom eye socket bone, right underneath the center of your eye. Press firmly with your two fingers for one second, then release for one second and repeat. Continue this for 30 seconds.

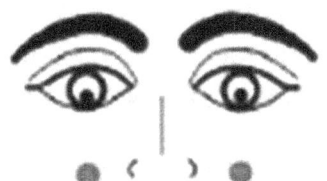

Example: press, release, press, release, press, release, etc.

Pinching the Bridge of the Nose

Close your eyes and place your thumb and pointer finger on either side of the bridge of your nose. Squeeze your finger and thumb together for one second, then release for one second, and repeat. Continue this for 30 seconds.

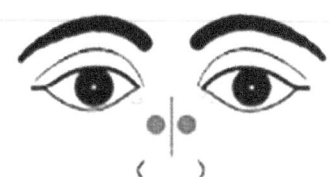

Example: squeeze, release, squeeze, release, squeeze, release, etc.

Combine all Acupressure Exercises Together

Combine all the above Acupressure exercises together to give your eyes a thorough massage. Start with Acupressure 1 for 30 seconds, then Acupressure 2 for 30 seconds, then Acupressure 3 for 30 seconds and then using your index and middle finger; gently tap in a circle around your entire eye socket. Start from Acupressure 1 position and work your way out and around the eye. Do this 3 times and then repeat, starting at Acupressure 1 for 30 seconds. Continue this cycle 5 times.

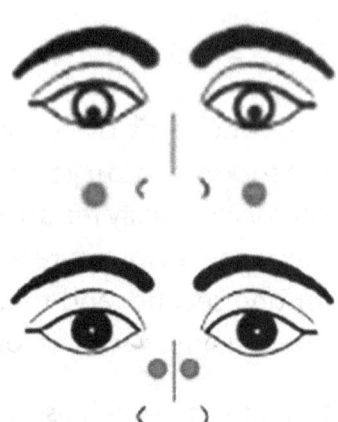

Example

Acupressure 1 – 30 seconds, Acupressure 2 – 30 seconds, Acupressure 3 – 30 seconds, tap around the eye – x3, Acupressure 1 – 30 seconds, Acupressure 2 – 30 seconds, Acupressure 3 – 30 seconds, tap around the eye – x3, etc.

Note: *Make sure to remove your glasses or contact lenses during exercises. If you want to work on maintaining a lower prescription, then wear your lowest prescription eyeglasses or contact lenses during the exercises.*

The following exercise routines should be done once a day and all in one sitting, for the full length of time. Do the eye exercise routines, in the order they appear in the chart.

It's important to do the exercise routines at a time throughout the day that you can relax and focus on the exercises. It's best to do them in the morning or before bed, to give your eyes the best chance at healing.

Make sure to take advantage of the bonus books with your order. Use the Success Journal and Eye Charts daily to monitor any progress with your vision.

IMPORTANT

If your eyes become sore or if you experience any headaches, slow down the exercises and use the eye strain exercises such as: Hydrotherapy, Slow Blink, Palming or Acupressure to relieve any stress.

Headaches and eyestrain are common side effects for the first two weeks of the eye exercises, however if they last more than a day (constant headache without breaks) or past 2 weeks, stop the exercises and see your doctor.

CHAPTER 10

EXERCISES FOR SPECIFIC EYE CONDITIONS

In this chapter I will show you the specialized eye routines for specific eye conditions. Remember, you can find out how to perform each of the exercises in the previous chapter.

The routines may take a little longer in the beginning while you learn the techniques, but once you know them, you'll fly through these exercises.

Remember if you ever have any questions regarding the exercises, just email support at *support@quantumvisionsys.com* and our highly trained team will be happy to help.

Note: *Make sure to remove your glasses or contact lenses during exercises. If you want to work on maintaining a lower prescription, then wear your lowest prescription eyeglasses or contact lenses during the exercises.*

Presbyopia & Hyperopia (Farsightedness)

Cause

Presbyopia is an eye condition where the lens of your eye loses its flexibility. This loss of flexibility makes it difficult to focus on close objects. Presbyopia is similar to Hyperopia, but is an age related eye condition that occurs around age 40, where the aging of the eye deteriorates the lens. Hyperopia (or Farsightedness) is an eye condition where distant objects appear clear, but close objects appear blurred. Hyperopia occurs when your eyeball is too short, or the cornea has too little curvature (opposite of Myopia). Too little curvature causes light entering the eye to not focus correctly on the retina.

Exercises

The goal of this exercise routine is to increase the nutrient flow in the eye and maximize flexibility of the inner lens. If you have Presbyopia or Hyperopia, you will benefit from the exercise routine below:

EXERCISE ROUTINE	TOTAL DURATION: 30 MINUTES
Palming	3 min
Eye Rolls	2 min
Clock Rotations	4 min
Squeeze Blinking	1 min
Pumping	2 min
Tromboning	2 min
Acupressure 4	5 min
Blur Zoning	3 min
Shifting	3 min
Hydrotherapy	5 min

Myopia (Nearsightewdness)

Cause

Myopia (or nearsightedness) is an eye condition where objects up close appear clear, but objects farther away appear blurred. This is caused when the eyeball or cornea is too long or has too much of a curvature. This over curvature causes light entering the eye to be unfocused on the retina, which sends the blurred vision to the brain through the optic nerve. Myopia can be caused by visual stress of doing too much work associated with close range vision, such as reading, or computer work. However adult myopia is usually caused by visual stress, as well as health conditions, such as diabetes.

Exercises

If you have Myopia (or nearsightedness), use the exercise routine below. On top of these exercises it is important to break any habits of reading up close, such as reading books, newspapers and using computers or laptops. Going outside and using your long-range vision is key. Playing certain long-range games such as golf, Frisbee, tennis or bowling could help cure your Myopia.

EXERCISE ROUTINE	TOTAL DURATION: 25 MINUTES
Palming	3 min
Pumping	2 min
Blur Zoning	3 min
Acupressure 4	5 min
Eye Rolls	2 min
Squeeze Blinking	2 min
Clock Rotations	3 min
Hydrotherapy	5 min

Astigmatism

Cause

Astigmatism is an eye condition that causes blurred vision at any distance. This is caused by an irregular shaped cornea or irregular curvature of the lens. Most people with Astigmatism have bad posture, and their head usually tilts towards a side. This causes the extraocular muscles of the eye to work overtime, by adjusting to the new vision, which is slightly tilted.

Exercises

This exercise routine is specifically designed for people with Astigmatism. You may find your eyes become sore after the exercises. If this occurs, follow up with the Eyestrain exercise routine to sooth your sore eyes.

Along with the exercises, it's important to correct the posture of your neck. To do this, place sticky notes angled in the opposite direction of your head tilt in various places around your home – your bathroom mirror, near the kitchen sink, on the pantry, on the wall near the bed, etc.

This will force you to tilt your head in the opposite direction every time you see the tilted sticky notes. Eventually your posture will improve automatically.

EXERCISE ROUTINE	TOTAL DURATION: 30 MINUTES
Palming	3 min
Eye Rolls	2 min
Clock Rotations	3 min
Acupressure 1	2 min
Eye Rolls	2 min
Clock Rotations	3 min
Acupressure 2	2 min
Eye Rolls	2 min

Clock Rotations	3 min
Acupressure 3	2 min
Squeeze Blinking	2 min
Slow Blinking	1 min
Hydrotherapy	3 min

Amblyopia & Strabismus (Lazy Eye & Crossed Eyes)

Cause

Amblyopia (or Lazy Eye) is the lack of development or loss of central vision in one eye. This is usually unrelated to any health problem and is not corrected using lenses. Amblyopia is caused by failure to use both eyes together. You will notice a lazy eye, by one eye always looking in a different direction compared to the good eye. Amblyopia is often associated with Strabismus (Crossed Eyes), which is an eye condition where both eyes do not look in the same direction at the same time. Strabismus is usually caused by poor extraocular muscles of the eye. Although you can usually notice a person with Amblyopia or Strabismus, it can be brought on by tired or strained eyes, excessive reading or computer work, or when the person is fighting an illness like a cold or flu.

Exercises

If you have a Lazy Eye or are Crossed Eyed, an eye patch over the dominant eye, usually the non-lazy eye, for several hours a day will help the weaker eye to develop. How to determine your dominant eye:

» Extend both your hands in front of your body, and create a small triangle by overlapping your thumbs and overlapping your fingers to the first knuckle.

» With both eyes open, look through the triangle and center an object in the middle – such as a doorknob (something small enough to fit into the triangle).

» Close your LEFT eye only – if the object remains in the triangle you are RIGHT eye dominant.

» Close your RIGHT eye only – if the object remains in the triangle you are LEFT eye dominant.

Once the weaker eye is working better, continue with the Myopia and Presbyopia/Hyperopia exercise routines. (Shown on the next page).

MYOPIA EXERCISE ROUTINE	TOTAL DURATION: 25 MINUTES
Palming	3 min
Pumping	3 min
Blur Zoning	3 min
Acupressure 4	5 min
Eye Rolls	2 min
Squeeze Blinking	2 min
Clock Rotation	1 min
Hydrotherapy	3 min

PRESBYOPIA/HYPEROPIA ROUTINE	TOTAL DURATION: 30 MINUTES
Palming	3 min
Eye Rolls	2 min
Clock Rotations	2 min
Squeeze Blinking	1 min
Pumping	3 min
Tromboning	3 min
Acupressure 4	5 min
Blur Zoning	3 min
Shifting	3 min
Hydrotherapy	5 min

Eye Floaters

Cause

Eye Floaters (or Spots) are small, cloudy, semi-transparent specks within the vitreous, which is the middle of the eye. Since they are inside your eye, they move when your eyes move, which is why they seem to dart away when you try to look directly at them. Eye Floaters are usually caused by small pieces of protein that were trapped in your eye during birth. They can also be caused by the deterioration of the vitreous fluid (fluid in the middle of the eye), due to aging of the eye. You can usually see Eye Floaters when your eyes are tired or strained.

Exercises

If you have Eye Floaters, use the exercise routine below. With this exercise routine we are trying to cleanse the eye and stimulate the flow of nutrients.

EXERCISE ROUTINE	TOTAL DURATION: 25 MINUTES
Palming	3 min
Pumping	2 min
Slow Blinking	1 min
Squeeze Blinking	1 min
Tromboning	2 min
Slow Blinking	1 min
Squeeze Blinking	1 min
Eye Rolls	2 min
Palming	3 min
Clock Rotations	2 min
Slow Blinking	1 min
Squeeze Blinking	1 min
Hydrotherapy	5 min

Dry Eye Syndrome (Keratoconjunctivitis Sicca (KCS))

Cause

Dry Eye Syndrome is an eye condition where there is insufficient tears to nourish the eye properly. Usually caused by poor production of tears or poor drainage.

Tears are a necessary part of maintaining the health of the cornea, which provides clear vision. They also reduce the risk of eye infection and can wash away foreign bodies from within the eye.

There are several factors that can cause Dry Eye Syndrome in people. Below is a list of the most common factors/causes:

» Medications – such as antihistamines, decongestants, antidepressants and blood pressure medications can reduce the production of tears in the eyes.

» Environmental Conditions – such as smoke, dry climates and wind can cause tear evaporation. Also excessive computer work, which causes a person to stare at the screen, can cause drying of the eyes.

» Contact Lenses – long-term use of contact lenses can cause your tear glands to malfunction and tear production to decrease. Dry eyes with contacts can also cause a bacterial infection or scratches on the cornea.

Exercises

Our main goal with this exercise routine is to encourage tear production in the eye. This exercise routine is designed specifically for people with Dry Eye Syndrome.

EXERCISE ROUTINE	TOTAL DURATION: 25 MINUTES
Hydrotherapy	3 min
Acupressure 1	2 min
Slow Blinking	2 min
Squeeze Blinking	2 min
Eye Rolls	2 min
Acupressure 2	2 min
Slow Blinking	2 min
Acupressure 3	2 min
Palming	5 min
Acupressure 4	3 min

Cataract

Cause

A normal eye consists of the eye's inner lens, which is made up of billions of living cells. Sometimes when we get older, these cells start to die which form a Cataract. A Cataract is simply the buildup of cellular debris (or dead cells). Below are some causes of Cataract:

» Ultraviolet light

» Toxic waste products

» Low nutrient levels in the body

Exercises

Our main focus with this exercise is to boost nutrient levels in the eye, while stimulating and cleansing the debris from the inner lens. If you have Cataracts, along with doing the exercise routine below, we recommend a balanced diet, which contains high amounts of Zinc, Vitamin E and Beta-Carotene. For more information on nourishing and cleansing your eyes, see Chapter 6.

EXERCISE ROUTINE	TOTAL DURATION: 25 MINUTES
Palming	3 min
Acupressure 1	2 min
Pumping	3 min
Acupressure 2	2 min
Tromboning	3 min
Acupressure 3	2 min
Eye Rolls	3 min
Acupressure 4	2 min
Hydrotherapy	5 min
Acupressure 4	3 min

Eyestrain

Cause

Stress especially on your eyes is an important issue to get fixed. If you do not fix eyestrain, it can seriously deteriorate the performance of your eye and ultimately cause vision problems.

Eyestrain or stress is usually brought on by focusing on something for a long period of time. Almost everyone stares at TV's, computers, and smartphones all day long. The light from the computer screen is causing your eyes to overwork. Especially your retina, which is constantly reflecting light.

This added stress causes symptoms such as:

» Headaches

» Eyelid tics or tension

» Dry eyes

» Bloodshot eyes

» Fatigue

» Loss of concentration

» Blurred or double vision (even with glasses)

Exercises

If you think you are suffering from eyestrain and have any of the above symptoms, try the exercise routine below:

EXERCISE ROUTINE	TOTAL DURATION: 25 MINUTES
Palming	5 min
Acupressure 4	5 min
Slow Blinking	5 min
Hydrotherapy	5 min
Palming	5 min

Macular Degeneration

Cause

Macular Degeneration is formed in a similar way to Cataracts. Although the eye exercises by themselves are not a cure for Macular degeneration, it will yield improvements. We recommend you use the Cataract eye exercise routine outlined below.

Exercises

These exercises will help bring nutrients to the back of the eye, where most of the problems lie. On top of the eye exercise routine, it's important to maintain a diet high in essential minerals and vitamins.

To speed up the healing process try taking 60mg of bilberry herbal extract per day, plus 5,000 mg of vitamin C and 500 mg of taurine (an amino acid). These supplements should be taken with food to avoid stomach irritation.

EXERCISE ROUTINE	TOTAL DURATION: 25 MINUTES
Palming	3 min
Acupressure 1	2 min
Pumping	3 min
Acupressure 2	2 min
Tromboning	3 min
Acupressure 3	2 min
Eye Rolls	3 min
Acupressure 4	2 min
Hydrotherapy	5 min

Glaucoma & EpiRetinal Membrane

Cause

Glaucoma is caused by fluid buildup in the eye, which can cause pressure to increase and can be extremely painful. EpiRetinal Membrane is a disease that is caused by changes in the fluid of the eye. With these eye conditions, it's important to work on improving the nutrients in the eye.

Exercises

These exercises will help bring nutrients to the back of the eye, where most of the problems lie. On top of the eye exercise routine, increasing your Vitamin A intake is an important part of healing Glaucoma. Try incorporating more carrots, cantaloupe, dried apricots, kale, sweet red peppers and/or sweet potatoes into your daily meals.

EXERCISE ROUTINE	TOTAL DURATION: 25 MINUTES
Palming	3 min
Pumping	3 min
Slow Blink	1 min
Tromboning	3 min
Palming	1 min
Eye Rolls	2 min
Slow Blink	1 min
Clock Rotations	3 min
Acupressure 4	3 min
Hydrotherapy	5 min

Keratoconus

Cause

Keratoconus is caused by changes in the fluid in the middle of the eye. Although the eye exercises by themselves are not a cure for Keratoconus, it will yield improvements. For this condition it's important to work on improving the nutrients in the eye.

Exercises

These exercises will help bring nutrients to the back of the eye.

EXERCISE ROUTINE	TOTAL DURATION: 25 MINUTES
Palming	3 min
Pumping	2 min
Slow Blink	1 min
Tromboning	2 min
Slow Blink	1 min
Clock Rotations	5 min
Palming	1 min
Eye Rolls	2 min
Acupressure 4	3 min
Hydrotherapy	5 min

DO YOU SUFFER FROM MORE THAN ONE EYE CONDITION LISTED ABOVE?

If you suffer from more than one eye condition, we recommend you alternate between the exercise routines. For example: Day 1 – Myopia exercise routine, Day 2 – Astigmatism exercise routine, Day 3 – Myopia, Day 4 – Astigmatism, etc.

The exercises should be done all in one sitting, for the full length of time. Do the eye exercise routines in the order they appear in the chart. Remember to do the exercise routines at a time throughout the day that you can relax and focus on the exercises. It's best to do them in the morning or before bed, to give your eyes the best chance at healing.

Maintenance: Seeing Results?

Once you are satisfied with the results you have achieved, we recommend slowing down the exercises, and only do the exercises 1 - 2 times a week.

If you have a specific eye condition that needs more attention (For example: Cataracts or Astigmatism), continue doing the specific eye exercise routine daily for at least 2 weeks, and then slowly decrease the times you preform the exercises (For example: 4 times a week, than 3 times a week, than 2 times a week, etc.)

Remember it's important to maintain a diet rich in vitamins and minerals, as it provides the right nutrients for your eyes to continue on their path of healing.

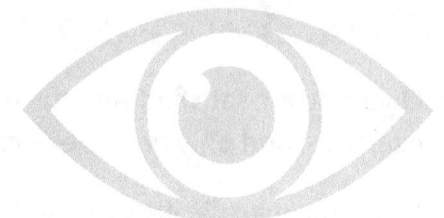

CHAPTER 11

BONUS: HEALING YOUR EYES WITH YOUR MIND

In the past decade or so, hundreds of studies have been conducted that demonstrate the powerful connection between mind and body. While Napoleon Hill figured it out many years ago, many scientists now believe that what you think about actually shapes your life.

For example, if you're constantly thinking about needing your glasses to see, your mind will automatically agree, causing you to have poor vision.

In landmark studies, Dr. Bruce Lipton proved that your mind can affect the cells of your body and even your DNA. It goes on to explain how our expectations and desires can affect our body's ability to fight illnesses and heal itself.

Now how do you use this "natural power" to heal your vision? Let's find out.

Is Your Subconscious Keeping You From Good Vision?

Each and every one of us has an image of ourselves in our subconscious mind. Your current self-image was built and shaped by interpretations and evaluations you place on past experiences.

For example, let's just say that at some time in your past, your eye doctor told you your vision was getting worse, or that you need to start wear glasses. And regardless of whether you noticed anything wrong with your vision, you may have started thinking there was. You may have imagined yourself being unable to see clearly. This may be something that you consciously or subconsciously played out in your mind.

Here's my point. It isn't the actual experience that shapes your self-image but the act of imagining yourself in a certain way that affects your self-image. Your mind and body react to your internal self-image. So, if your self-image is that of a person with poor vision, your body will do everything that it can to make that true.

As I've said earlier, current scientific research actually shows that your mind affects the cells of your body and even your DNA. So if your self-image is someone with poor vision, your cells will actually force you to see poorly. Your self-image has a powerful effect on your body.

In order to be glasses free, you need to change your self-image. Luckily, there's an easy way to do this.

21-Day Visualization Exercises

The mind is a powerful thing to waste. And wherever the mind goes, the body will follow. Harnessing the power of our mind is so powerful and yet very few of us actually use its power to shape our self-image and to create perfect health.

The first thing to do is to get a clear image in your mind's eye of what it would feel like to be glasses free, the ideal you.

Begin by imagining yourself completely free of glasses or contact lenses. Free of blurred vision. Imagine going to your optometrist and to their amazement, you're vision actually reversed course and now you have perfect 20/20 vision.

I promise you, if you give this an honest effort, you'll be so thrilled with the results and you'll choose to continue using this tool for the rest of your life.

We have purposely asked you to challenge yourself for three weeks, as research has proven that it takes 21 days to make a substantial change to your self-image.

As I've said before, your current self-image was created by your imagination. So we can use this same method to create a new self-image where you enjoy your perfect, healthy body.

Remember, all you have to do is sit back, relax and imagine yourself as you wish to be. Here's how:

1 Grab a piece of paper and write a brief description of the image that you intend to view in your mind. This will be the movie you will play over in your mind.

2 Every day, find a quiet place where you won't be disturbed. Now, close your eyes and begin playing the movie you wrote down in your mind for at least 20 minutes.

3 For the first 7 days, refine your movie to picture your body exactly as you desire it to be. Then, for the remaining 14 days, play this exact movie in your mind over and over again.

HERE ARE SOME TIPS TO MAKE THIS VISUALIZATION TECHNIQUE MORE EFFECTIVE

TIP

» Most people find that they get better results if they imagine themselves sitting at a theatre and watching themselves as the star character in the movie on the big screen.

» It's important to make your mental movie of yourself as vivid and detailed as possible to stimulate actual experiences. For example, instead of just picturing your body being healthy, imagine your eyes repairing and your vision improving every day. Imagine how you would feel to be glasses free.

» Pay attention to the small details. The more detailed, the more your subconscious will believe it to be an actual experience. Make sure to use all your senses.

» It's important to see yourself as you want to be. It doesn't matter where your health is today. You need to have faith in this exercise.

CHAPTER 12
CONCLUSION

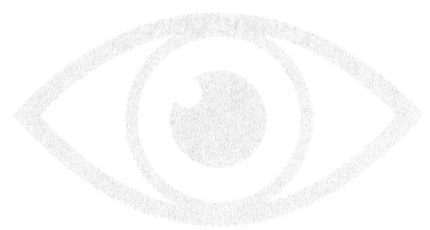

Seeing clearly without glasses or contact lenses, shouldn't just be for the lucky few. It's a right that everyone should have, even you!

Imagine waking up each day and not having to reach for your glasses or stumble to the bathroom to put in your contact lenses.

Imagine waking up, walking to the kitchen and seeing your family's smiling faces! This can and will happen to you.

Cleanse and nourish your eyes, take the nutritional supplements, do the Quantum Vision Exercises and imagine your vision get better each day.

I promise, if you commit to make these changes, you will be thrilled with the results!

I can't wait to hear from you. Don't forget to send me a quick email or video testimonial letting us know your progress and how the Quantum Vision System has helped you. Testimonials help others have the confidence to restore their vision too.

If you have any questions or concerns about the system, I encourage you to email our support team at *support@quantumvisionsys.com*.

And remember, if you aren't 100% satisfied with this system, you are backed by our 60-day money back guarantee. Simply let us know and we'll refund your money, no questions asked!

Again, thank you for taking the chance on the Quantum Vision System and believing in the Truth! Remember to stay positive and enjoy your glasses-free life!

Quantum Vision System 3-Step Recap

STEP 1

Optimize Your Diet & Cleanse

» Eat a nutrient rich diet the human body was designed for

» Cleanse your body and eyes from chemicals and pollutants

STEP 2

Nourish Your Eyes

» Add compounds that reverse & repair damaged eye cells

» Supplement key nutrients your eyes need for optimal sight

STEP 3

Eye Strengthening Exercises

» Follow the daily Quantum Vision Exercises to restore your vision naturally

» Have an eye condition? Cure it naturally with a specific eye exercise routine

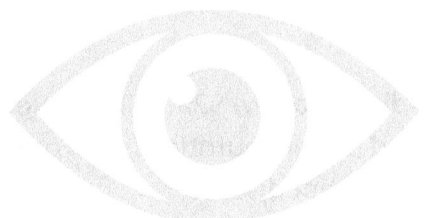

CHAPTER 13
RECIPES

As you move forward with the Quantum Vision System, it's vital that you have a small number of recipes so that you can become healthy and still eat great. It's always easier to stick to a new eating plan when meals are more satisfying.

You can try something new every day, week or month. Start adding these easy, mouth-watering food recipes and watch for fantastic results.

Whole Foods

When it comes to eating, it's all about quality over quantity. And eating quality food means that you are eating whole foods.

What is a whole food?

Well, as I hope you've learned in the previous chapters, our bodies run best on a natural diet that is free of food that has been manufactured or altered. I'm talking about junk food, processed food and grains, artificially sweetened products, fried foods, and what we know as the Standard American Diet.

These foods were created in laboratories by chemists and our bodies do not know how to digest these chemical, hybrid foods.

A whole food is an apple, some berries, a whole grain such as quinoa or brown rice, and even a piece of fish. This is the way that nature intends us to eat. And if this sounds at all overwhelming, don't worry. All of the recipes use these whole foods and are easy to prepare.

Go Organic

Whenever possible, buy organic fruits and vegetables. According to a new $25-million study into organic food – the largest of its kind to date – organic food is more nutritious than ordinary produce and it may help to lengthen people's lives and prevent disease.

The study found that organic fruit and vegetables have up to 50% more antioxidants, which scientists believe can cut the risk of cancer and heart disease. Organic produce also has more vitamins and minerals such as iron and zinc. Not to mention the taste of organic fruits and vegetables is often superior to any conventional produce.

The Quantum Vision Diet

It's critically important that you eat more fruit and vegetables, especially raw. You can also eat good fats and meat in moderations. Basically, you'll be eating real food; the food nature intended us to eat.

Once you've restored your vision, you may begin to introduce a few more foods. Don't go crazy on junk. Remember, it's what caused the problem in the first place.

So, what are you waiting for? Let's get started.

Salad Dressings

Basic Salad Dressing

 INGREDIENTS

¼ cup red wine vinegar

½ cup extra virgin olive oil

1 tsp. sea salt

 INSTRUCTIONS

- Put all ingredients in a jar and shake to combine.

Asian Salad Dressing

 INGREDIENTS

3 tbsp. extra virgin olive oil

3 tbsp. cider vinegar

1 tbsp. soy sauce

1 tsp. toasted sesame oil

1 tsp. sesame seeds

1 garlic clove, minced

¼ tsp. sea salt

¼ tsp. pepper

INSTRUCTIONS

- Put all ingredients in a jar and shake to combine.

Greek Dressing

 ## INGREDIENTS

2 small garlic cloves, minced

½ tsp. Dijon mustard

1 tsp. dried oregano

3 tbsp. apple cider vinegar

Juice of ½ lemon

½ cup extra virgin olive oil

¾ tsp. sea salt

½ tsp. black pepper

 ## INSTRUCTIONS

- Put all ingredients in a jar and shake to combine. For best results, let sit for 30 minutes to deepen flavors.

Avocado and Cilantro Dressing

 ## INGREDIENTS

1 large avocado

½ bunch of fresh cilantro

Juice of 4 juicy limes

¼ cup extra virgin olive oil

1 clove garlic, minced

Salt and pepper to taste

 ## INSTRUCTIONS

- Mix all ingredients in a blender or a big bowl (with a little elbow grease).
- Season to taste.

Creamy Caesar Salad Dressing

INGREDIENTS

1 egg yolk

1 tbsp. Dijon mustard

½ cup extra virgin olive oil

2 cloves garlic

4 anchovy fillets

1 tsp. black pepper

1 lemon, juiced

INSTRUCTIONS

- Combine all ingredients except for olive oil in a food processor.
- Once smooth, slowly add oil until everything is emulsified.

Ginger Tamari Garlic Dressing

INGREDIENTS

¼ cup flax oil

⅛ cup apple cider vinegar

⅛ cup gluten-free tamari or Bragg's liquid seasoning

1 small clove garlic, minced very fine

1.5 tsp. fresh ginger, minced very fine

INSTRUCTIONS

- Combine all ingredients in a jar and shake to combine.

Ultra Creamy Hemp Dressing

INGREDIENTS

½ cup hulled hemp seeds

½ cup water

2 tbsp. nutritional yeast

2 tbsp. fresh lemon juice

1 clove garlic, peeled

½ tsp. fine grain sea salt

INSTRUCTIONS

- Add all dressing ingredients to a high-speed blender and blend on high until smooth.

- Adjust salt to taste.

- The dressing will appear thin at first but will thicken up after being chilled in the fridge.

Salads

Basic Salad

INGREDIENTS

6 cups mixed greens

1 carrot, grated

1 cup red cabbage, thinly sliced

1 cup cherry tomatoes, cut in half

¼ red onion, sliced

INSTRUCTIONS

- Combine all ingredients in a large bowl. When ready to serve, top with dressing.

Beet Salad

INGREDIENTS

1 beet, grated

4 cups mixed greens

2 tbsp. minced fresh parsley

½ lemon, juiced

2 tbsp. extra virgin olive oil or flax oil

Sea salt and pepper

INSTRUCTIONS

- Divide mixed greens among two plates. Top with grated beet and apple.
- Whisk lemon juice and oil in a bowl.
- Season with a little salt and pepper and drizzle overtop of the salad.
- Finally, sprinkle minced parsley overtop and serve.

Asian Coleslaw

INGREDIENTS

1 small head of cabbage, thinly sliced

4 green onions, sliced

1 carrot, grated or cut into matchsticks

1 tbsp. sesame seeds

INSTRUCTIONS

- Combine all ingredients in a bowl and top with Ginger Tamari Garlic Dressing. This salad gets better after it has marinated for at least 30 minutes.

Kale Caesar Salad

- -

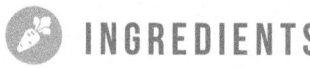 **INGREDIENTS**

1 head of kale, washed

½ lemon, juiced

1 quantity Caesar Dressing

INSTRUCTIONS

- Thoroughly dry the kale. Remove from the large stem and tear into bite-sized pieces.

- Place kale pieces in a large bowl and add lemon juice. Massage the lemon juice into the kale until it begins to wilt.

- Pour over dressing and mix to combine. Place in the refrigerator for at least one hour before serving.

Vegetable Dishes

Steamed Asparagus

- -

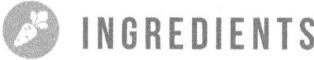 **INGREDIENTS**

1 pound fresh asparagus, ends trimmed

1 lemon, juiced

Fresh parsley, chopped

Salt and pepper

INSTRUCTIONS

- Wash the asparagus and cut into 2" pieces.

- Fill a medium-sized saucepan halfway with water and bring to a boil.

- Add the asparagus and reduce heat to a simmer for 2 minutes.

- Drain asparagus, put in a bowl and top with lemon juice, parsley, salt and pepper.

Cauliflower Rice

 INGREDIENTS

1 clove garlic, minced

1 tbsp. coconut oil

½ head cauliflower

Sea salt and pepper

 INSTRUCTIONS

- Rinse cauliflower under cool water and pat dry.
- Using a cheese grater, grate the cauliflower to a coarse texture (approximately the size of rice grains). (Using a food processor to pulse the cauliflower to desired texture also works.)
- Heat the coconut oil in a skillet over medium heat.
- Sauté the garlic for 1-2 minutes.
- Add in the cauliflower rice and continue to sauté for 4 - 5 minutes.
- Season with salt and pepper, and serve.

Stir-Fried Garlicky Swiss Chard

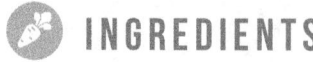 **INGREDIENTS**

1 bunch Swiss chard

3 cloves garlic, sliced

1 tbsp. extra-virgin olive oil

2-3 tbsp. water

Pinch red pepper flakes

Sea salt and pepper

INSTRUCTIONS

- Wash and dry the chard. Trim the thick stems and slice into ½" pieces as you would with celery.

- Slice the leaves into 1" strips.

- Heat the oil in a pan over medium heat and add the stems. Cook until the stems begin to soften, around five minutes.

- Add chard to the pan. Put the sliced garlic and chili flakes overtop and sprinkle a few tablespoons of water into the pan.

- Stir-fry until the chard wilts. Season lightly with salt and pepper and serve.

Roasted Brussels Sprouts

INGREDIENTS

1 ½ pounds Brussels Sprouts

2 tbsp. coconut oil (warm it up to
melt it)

¾ tsp. sea salt

½ tsp. pepper

INSTRUCTIONS

- Preheat the oven to 400 °F.

- Cut off the brown ends of the sprouts and remove yellow outer leaves.

- Mix in a bowl with oil, salt and pepper. Lay out on a baking pan and place in the oven for 30-35 minutes.

- Shake the sprouts from time to time to ensure that everything browns evenly.

Broccoli with Toasted Almonds

INGREDIENTS

1 bunch broccoli, cut into bite-sized florets, stems peeled and cut into quarters

¼ cup almonds

INSTRUCTIONS

- Add 1" of water to a medium saucepan. Cover with a steamer and bring to a boil. Add broccoli to steamer and cook until tender, around 5-6 minutes.

- Meanwhile, put almonds in a pan heated to medium heat and toast until fragrant, 1-2 minutes. Remove to cutting board and roughly chop.

- Serve broccoli in a large bowl, with almonds scattered overtop.

Protein Dishes

Broccoli, Bacon and Egg Bake

🥕 INGREDIENTS

4 slices organic bacon

8 eggs

½ large onion, diced

2 medium zucchini, diced

1 cup broccoli, chopped

1 tsp. sea salt

½ tsp. pepper

1 tbsp. fresh parsley, chopped

🍲 INSTRUCTIONS

- Preheat oven to 350 °F.
- In a skillet, cook the bacon until cooked through. Reserve to a paper towel and cut into small strips.
- Wipe away most of the fat from the skillet, leaving around 1 tbsp. Add the onion and sauté for 3 minutes. Add zucchini and broccoli and sauté until they have softened a bit. Remove from heat.
- In a bowl, whisk the eggs with the salt and pepper.
- Grease a baking dish (must be large enough to hold the eggs and vegetables) with coconut oil. Add the vegetables.
- Pour over egg mixture and bake 25-30 minutes or until the eggs are set.

Perfect Roast Chicken with Leeks

🥕 INGREDIENTS

1 4lbs. chicken, rinsed, and patted dry

½ bunch thyme

½ bunch rosemary

2 leeks, halved and rinsed well

1 tsp. extra virgin olive oil

Sea salt and pepper

INSTRUCTIONS

- Preheat oven to 450 °F. Season chicken inside and out with salt and pepper and place in a roasting pan. Stuff thyme and rosemary in cavity.

- In a large bowl, toss leeks with oil; season with salt and pepper.

- Scatter leeks around chicken. Roast until chicken is golden brown and juices run clear when pierced between breast and leg (an instant-read thermometer inserted in thickest part of a thigh, avoiding bone, should read 165 degrees), about 1 hour.

Pesto Chicken and Tomato Kebabs

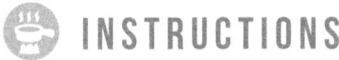

INGREDIENTS

1 cup fresh basil leaves, chopped

1 clove garlic

1 ¼ lbs. skinless chicken breast, cut into 1" cubes

24 cherry tomatoes

16 wooden skewers

Salt and pepper, to taste

INSTRUCTIONS

- In a food processor, pulse basil, garlic and salt and pepper until smooth.

- Combine the raw chicken with pesto and marinate a few hours in the fridge. Soak wooden skewers in water at least 30 minutes (or use metal ones to avoid this step).

- Beginning and ending with chicken, thread the chicken and tomatoes onto 8 pairs of parallel skewers to make 8 kebabs total.

- Heat an outdoor grill or grill pan over medium heat. Place the chicken on the grill and cook around 3-4 minutes on each side.

- Serve and enjoy!

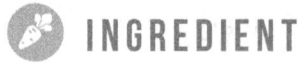

Grilled Chicken with Spinach

INGREDIENTS

21 oz. (3 large) chicken breasts, sliced in half lengthwise to make 6 cutlets

Salt and pepper to taste

3 cloves garlic, crushed

10 oz. frozen spinach, drained

1 red bell pepper, chopped

INSTRUCTIONS

- Season chicken with salt and pepper. Grill on an outdoor grill or grill pan until cooked through.

- Meanwhile, heat a sauté pan over medium heat. Add bell pepper, garlic, spinach and some salt and pepper. Cook until heated throughout.

- To serve, top each piece of chicken with the spinach and pepper mixture. Enjoy!

Tuna Salad in Red Pepper Boats

INGREDIENTS

1 can light tuna in water

¼ cup celery, chopped

¼ cup red onion, chopped

¼ cup broccoli florets

½ lemon, juiced

1 tbsp. extra-virgin olive oil

½ tsp. dried dill or 1 tsp. fresh dill

Fresh ground pepper

1 red pepper, cut into quarters

INSTRUCTIONS

- Drain tuna. Mix all ingredients except for peppers in a bowl. Serve by scooping tuna mixture into red pepper boats.

Easy Baked Italian Fish

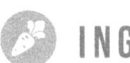 **INGREDIENTS**

1 large fillet (or two small) white fish, such as whitefish, halibut or cod

8 cloves garlic

8 kalmata olives, pitted

1 tbsp. capers (optional)

1 pint cherry tomatoes

Drizzle of extra virgin olive oil

Sea salt and pepper

2 lemon wedges

4 big handfuls arugula or spinach

Handful roughly torn Italian parsley

 INSTRUCTIONS

- Preheat the oven to 350 °F. Drizzle olive oil in a baking dish and place fish on baking dish. Arrange tomatoes, capers, olives and garlic.

- Sprinkle a pinch of sea salt and a grind of pepper overtop and place in the oven.

- Bake until fish is flaky and tomatoes are about to burst, around 10-15 minutes.

- Divide arugula or spinach among two plates. Top each with half the fish, tomatoes, garlic, olives and capers if using. Sprinkle some parsley overtop, serve with a lemon wedge and an extra pinch of sea salt and pepper.

Salmon with Tomato Salsa

 ## SALMON INGREDIENTS

4 salmon fillets

Salt and pepper

 ## SALSA INGREDIENTS

3 medium tomatoes, diced

1 lime, juiced

¼ red onion, diced

¼ cup cilantro, chopped

1 garlic clove, finely chopped

Salt and pepper

 ## INSTRUCTIONS

- Preheat the oven to 350°F. Sprinkle salt and pepper over salmon. Bake in the oven for 10-12 minutes, or until the salmon flakes with fork.

- Meanwhile, mix all salsa ingredients in a bowl and stir to combine.

- To serve, top each piece of salmon with the salsa mixture.

Bunless Salmon Burgers

 ## INGREDIENTS

1 (1-pound) salmon fillet, skinned and chopped

2 cups chopped baby spinach

¼ cup panko (Japanese breadcrumbs)

1 tbsp. fresh lemon juice

1 tbsp. finely grated fresh ginger

1 tbsp. low-sodium soy sauce

¼ cup sesame seeds, toasted and divided

¼ tsp. salt

¼ tsp. black pepper

½ tsp. minced garlic

Olive oil

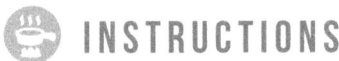

INSTRUCTIONS

- Combine salmon, spinach, panko, 1 tbsp. lemon juice, ginger, soy sauce, garlic, 1 tbsp. sesame seeds, salt, and pepper in a large bowl. Form mixture into 4 (3 1/2-inch) patties. Place remaining sesame seeds onto a plate, and dip one side of patties into seeds to coat.

- Preheat a lightly oiled grill pan over medium heat until hot but not smoking. Cook burgers over medium heat, turning, 3-4 minutes per side or until golden brown and cooked through.

- Serve on pieces of lettuce with sliced onion and tomato. Poached Eggs Over Garlicky Greens

Poached Eggs Over Garlicky Greens

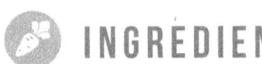 INGREDIENTS

2 eggs

1 tbsp. extra-virgin olive oil

4 cups spinach or ½ bunch kale or

Swiss chard

2 cloves garlic

Salt and pepper to taste

INSTRUCTIONS

- To poach the eggs, fill a saucepan with a couple inches of water. Heat the water on high until it reaches a bare simmer and bubbles start appearing at the bottom of the pan.

- Crack each egg into a small bowl or cup. Place the bowl close to the surface of the hot water and gently slip the egg into the water. Turn off the heat and cover the pan.

- Set a timer for 4 minutes. At this point the egg whites should be completely cooked, while the egg yolks are still runny. Gently lift the poached eggs out of the pan with a slotted spoon and place on a plate to serve.

- Meanwhile, heat the olive oil in a sauté pan over medium heat. Add garlic and as much spinach as you can fit in the pan. (It will wilt and reduce in size.) Keep adding spinach and letting it wilt.

- To serve, spoon greens into a bowl and top with poached eggs and a sprinkle of salt and pepper.

Meatloaf

🥕 INGREDIENTS

1 lb. extra lean ground beef

½ onion, finely chopped

1 tbsp. chili powder

2 tbsp. Worcestershire sauce

1 egg

2 tbsp. Dijon mustard

🍳 INSTRUCTIONS

- Preheat oven to 400 °F. Crumble ground beef into a large bowl.

- Add chopped onion and green pepper. Add chili powder, Worcestershire sauce and Dijon mustard. Stir with fork. Add egg and stir again until well mixed.

- You may knead the mixture with your hands but take care not to over mix (this will make the meat tough).

- Spoon the mixture into an oiled muffin pan. Bake for 25 minutes, making sure that the internal temperature reaches 165°F.

Roasted Flank Steak with Herbs

INGREDIENTS

1 tsp. fresh thyme, chopped

1 tsp. fresh oregano, chopped

1 tsp. fresh parsley, chopped

⅛ tsp. grated lemon rind

1 garlic clove, minced

½ tsp. salt

¼ tsp. freshly ground black pepper

1 ½ lb. flank steak, trimmed

Thyme sprigs, optional

🍳 INSTRUCTIONS

- Preheat oven to 400 °F. Combine thyme, oregano, parsley, lemon rind and garlic in a small bowl. Set aside.

- Sprinkle salt and pepper over steak. Heat a large ovenproof skillet over medium-high heat. Add steak and cook 1 minute on each side or until browned.

- Spread herb mixture over steak and place pan in oven. Bake for 10 minutes or until cooked to your liking.

- Let stand 10 minutes before cutting steak diagonally across the grain into thin slices. Serve with pan sauce, garnish with fresh thyme sprigs, if desired.

Garlic Lime Marinated Pork Chops

 ## INGREDIENTS

4 (6 oz. each) lean boneless pork chops

4 cloves garlic, crushed

1 tsp. cumin

1 tsp. chili powder

1 tsp. paprika

½ lime, juiced

Lime zest

Salt and pepper, to taste

 ## INSTRUCTIONS

- Trim any fat off pork. In a large bowl, season pork with garlic, cumin, chili powder, paprika, salt and pepper. Squeeze lime juice and some zest from the lime and let it marinate at least 20 minutes.

- Place pork chops on a broiler pan and broil 4-5 minutes on each side or until nicely browned.

Summer Vegetables with Sausage

🥕 INGREDIENTS

14 oz. Italian sausage, with no added sugar, sliced 1" thick

1 large onion, chopped

Salt and pepper, to taste

4-5 cloves garlic, smashed with side of knife

½ orange bell pepper, diced into 1" squares

½ yellow pepper, diced into 1" squares

1 red bell pepper, diced into 1" squares

2 tbsp. fresh rosemary (or other fresh herb such as thyme)

2 cups zucchini, ½" thick and quartered

🍳 INSTRUCTIONS

- Add sausage to the skillet and sauté over medium-low heat, stirring occasionally until browned but not quite cooked through, about10 minutes.

- Season chopped vegetables with salt and pepper. Add onions, peppers, garlic and rosemary to the skillet and mix.

- Continue cooking, stirring occasionally until onions and peppers become slightly browned. Add zucchini and cook an additional 5 minutes, mixing until everything is cooked.

Shepherd's Pie

INGREDIENTS

1 head cauliflower, chopped into florets

2 tbsp. coconut oil

1 small onion, diced

2 celery ribs, diced

2 carrots, diced

2 cloves garlic, minced

1 pound ground beef or lamb

¼ - ½ cup homemade beef broth

1 tbsp. tomato paste

2 tbsp. chopped parsley

Salt and pepper to taste

2 tbsp. coconut oil

INSTRUCTIONS

- Preheat the oven to 400 °F. Grease a 2-3 quart casserole dish and set aside.

- In a large pot, steam or boil cauliflower until tender.

- Heat 2 tbsp. of fat in a large skillet or saucepan over medium high heat. Add the onion, celery, carrots and garlic and cook until beginning to soften, around 5 minutes.

- Add the ground meat to the pan and cook until browned. Add beef broth as necessary to keep the mixture wet. Add the ketchup or tomato paste (if using), parsley and season with salt and pepper. Let simmer while you prepare the cauliflower topping.

- To make the topping, drain the cooked cauliflower. Mash or puree with a stick blender until smooth. Add 2 tbsp. of fat and season with salt and pepper.

- To assemble, spread the meat mixture on the bottom of the dish. Top with the cauliflower mixture and smooth with a spoon. Cover with shredded cheese, if using.

- Bake for 30 minutes or until the top is brown and bubbly. Serve warm.

Grilled Rosemary Lamb Chops

INGREDIENTS

4 lean lamb chops

3 cloves garlic, crushed

¼ cup fresh lemon juice

1 tbsp. fresh rosemary leaves

Salt and pepper, to taste

INSTRUCTIONS

- Combine lemon juice, garlic and rosemary. Season the lamb with salt and pepper and cover with garlic mixture.

- Marinate at least 1 hour, overnight if possible. Discard the marinade, then grill or broil over medium-high heat to desired liking.

Turkey Taco Lettuce Wraps

INGREDIENTS

1.3 lbs. 99% lean ground turkey

1 tsp. garlic powder

1 tsp. cumin

1 tsp. salt

1 tsp. chili powder

1 tsp. paprika

½ tsp. oregano

½ small onion, minced

2 tbsp. bell pepper, minced

¾ cup water

4 oz. can tomato sauce

8 large leaves from iceberg lettuce

INSTRUCTIONS

- Brown turkey in a large skillet, breaking it into smaller pieces as it cooks. When it is no longer pink, add dry seasonings and mix well.

- Add the onion, pepper, water and tomato sauce and cover. Simmer on low for about 20 minutes.

- Wash and dry the lettuce. Divide the meat equally between the 8 leaves and enjoy.

BBQ Ribs

 ### INGREDIENTS

4 lbs. baby back pork ribs

Salt and pepper to taste

Cayenne pepper

Garlic powder

 ### INSTRUCTIONS

- Place ribs on a large sheet of heavy-duty aluminum foil and rub on all sides with the salt, pepper, cayenne and garlic powder. Preheat grill for high heat.

- Place ribs in foil on the grill grate and cook 1 hour. Remove ribs from foil and place directly on grill gate. Continue cooking 30 minutes until ribs are done.

Zucchini "Spaghetti" with Meatballs

INGREDIENTS

MEATBALLS

1 tbsp. coconut oil (for frying)

2 medium eggs

1 pound ground beef

½ cup almond meal or coconut flour

2 tbsp. nutritional yeast

1 clove garlic, minced

1 tsp. Italian seasoning

2 tsp. tamari or soy sauce

1 tsp. oregano

1 tsp. sea salt

¼ tsp. red pepper flakes

SAUCE

1 jar organic pasta sauce

"NOODLES"

4 large zucchinis

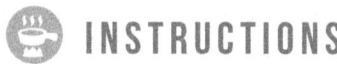

INSTRUCTIONS

MEATBALLS

- Whisk the eggs in the bottom of a big bowl. Add the remaining ingredients. Knead the mixture with your hands until everything is just mixed. Form the meat into golf ball-sized meatballs.

- Heat the olive oil in a large dutch-oven or heavy-bottomed pot over medium heat. Pan fry the meatballs in batches, until browned all over. They do not need to cook all the way through since they will simmer in the sauce.

- Add the meatballs to the sauce and simmer over medium heat for 20 minutes, until the meatballs are cooked through and the sauce is thickened. Stir occasionally.

"NOODLES"

- Lay the first zucchini on a cutting board. Cut off both ends.

- With a vegetable peeler, peel along the length of the zucchini. Discard the peel and continue peeling. Stack the pieces as you go. Stop once you hit the seeds and rotate. Continue on all sides.

- Repeat with remaining zucchinis.

- Take a few slices of zucchini and lay them on top of one another. Cut lengthwise into "noodles."

- Repeat with remaining pieces of zucchini.

- Toss the noodles into a bowl and sprinkle salt overtop. Mix to combine. Place the zucchini into a colander so that the water in the zucchini can drip out. Wait 20 minutes and then rinse.

- Pat dry with a paper towel.

- To serve, divide noodles among 4 plates. Top with sauce and meatballs and serve!

BONUS
EYE CHARTS

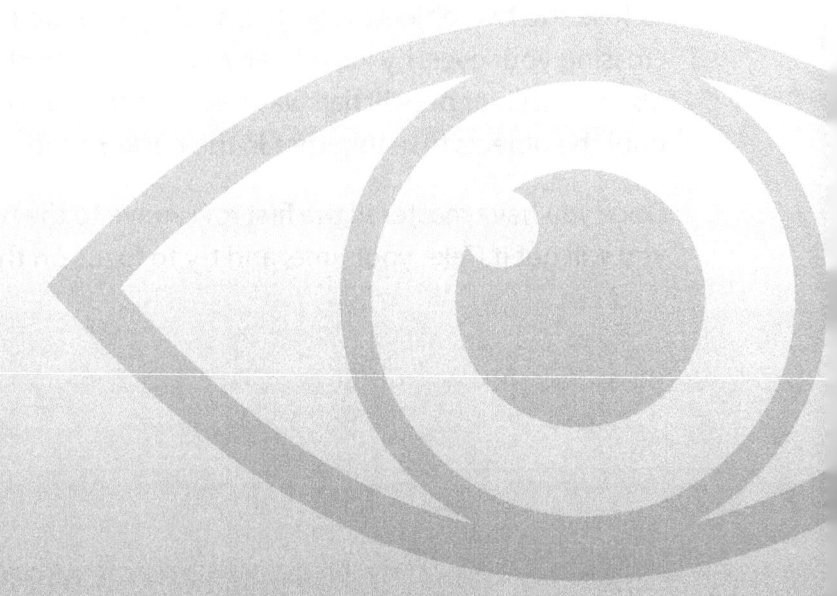

THE USE OF CHARTS

Introduction

Eye charts are a great way to improve your eyes extraocular muscles and to work on improving your astigmatism, nearsightedness or farsightedness. Think of these eye chart exercises as a turbo boost to improving your vision. Include these eye charts with your Quantum Vision Exercises, eating right and your daily visualized healing and you will be seeing 20/20 in no time.

We've included all the charts at the back of this book for easy use. We recommend you tear off the pages the charts are on and use them daily.

Note: Remember to rest your eyes after each exercise below. Use Palming or Slow Blinking (or a combination of the two) between exercises to relax your eye muscles.

Note: Make sure to remove your glasses or contact lenses during exercises. If you want to work on maintaining a lower prescription, then wear your lowest prescription eyeglasses or contact lenses during the exercises.

Fusion Chart

The Fusion Chart works your extraocular muscles. This trains your extraocular muscles to work as a team.

Hold the Fusion Chart arm's length away from your face. Stare at the top row of circles. Try to fuse the two objects together, so they overlap each other. If you are having trouble, try crossing your eyes, by looking at your nose, then slowly uncross them. Or you can place an object (a pen or pencil) half way between the Fusion Chart and your eyes. Focus on the pen until the objects fuse together in the background.

Once you have mastered the first row, move to the next one. It takes practice, but eventually you will get it. Take your time, and try to focus on the outline of the object.

Fusion Pumping

Fusion pumping works your extraocular muscles and also helps increase the flow of nutrients while exercising the focusing mechanisms of the eye.

Once you feel comfortable fusing the objects in all rows of the Fusion Chart, you can try Fusion Pumping. Just like regular Pumping, you will be focusing your vision on a near object and then a far object. Alternating between the two. But for this exercise you will be using the Fusion Chart as your near object. Every time you look at the Fusion Chart, fuse the first row objects together. Once they have overlapped, look at a far object. Continue with the first row 5 times. Then move onto the next row for 5 times, and so on until you have finished the Fusion Chart.

Scanning Chart

The Scanning Chart is similar to Blur Zoning, as it helps work on your eyes ability to see detail. Eventually helping to restore your vision.

Place the large Scanning Chart just in your blur zone so it is slightly blurred. If you are Myopia (Nearsighted) – hold the chart in front of your face, if you are Hyperopia (Farsighted) – tape the chart on a wall. Looking at the chart, jump your eyes from dot to dot (similar to Shifting) and follow the lines from Start to Finish. Then go backwards from Finish to Start. Make sure to focus on each dot for a couple of seconds, before moving to the next dot.

Next use the small Scanning Chart. You will need to move this chart closer to you. Place it just in your blur zone where the chart becomes slightly blurry. Start at the Start line and begin jumping from one dot to the next, until you have reached the Finish line. Then go backwards from Finish to Start. Again make sure to focus on each dot for a couple of seconds, before moving onto the next dot.

Repeat this exercise a couple of times, from Start to Finish, and then Finish to Start. Each time you start over, change the position of the chart, so that your eyes don't get familiar with the path. Example: rotate the image to the right or left, or hold it upside down.

Once the Scanning Charts become too easy, place the chart deeper in your blur zone. Congratulations, this means you are improving your vision!

Acuity Chart

The Acuity Chart is similar to the Scanning Chart, as it works on your eyes ability to see detail.

Place the Acuity Chart just in your blur zone. Look at the smallest line you can read. Slowly look over the words, see if you can read any of them. Then take a word, and slowly focus on the outline of the word. Make sure to stay calm and breath, there is no rush. Don't squint or stare at the word. Blink frequently and constantly look around the outline of the word. Once you can make out 2 or 3 words on the line, move to the next smallest line. Continue this exercise until you can make out words on every line. Then move the chart further into your blur zone. Hooray! You are improving your vision.

Conclusion

Continue with these exercises until you start to see improvements. Remember to always give your eyes a rest in-between exercises using Palming, Slow Blinking or Hydrotherapy. Don't forget to send support (*support@quantumvisionsys.com*) an email or video on your progress. We can't wait to hear about your vision improvements.

Fusion Chart

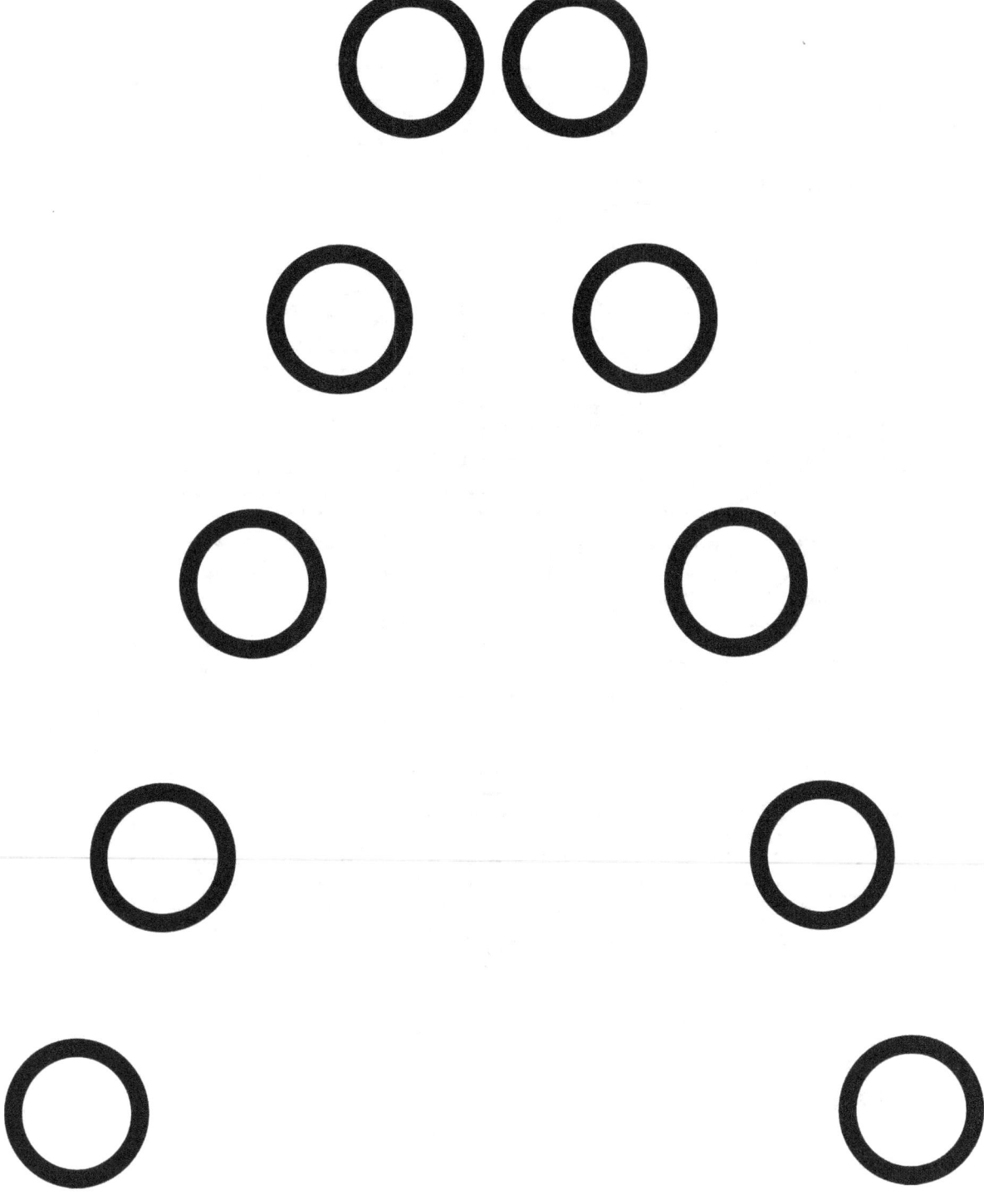

Scanning Chart (Large)

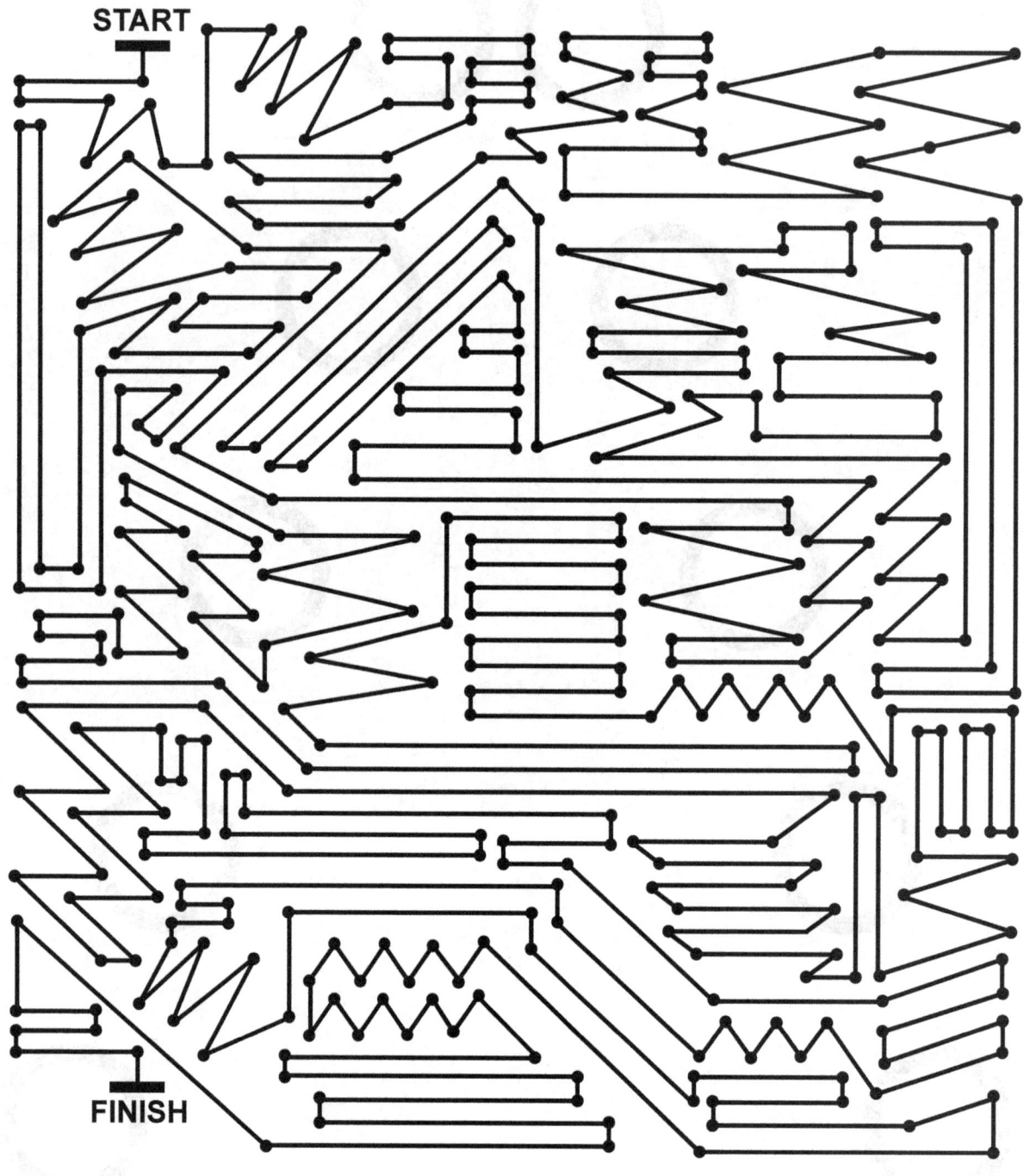

Scanning Chart (Small)

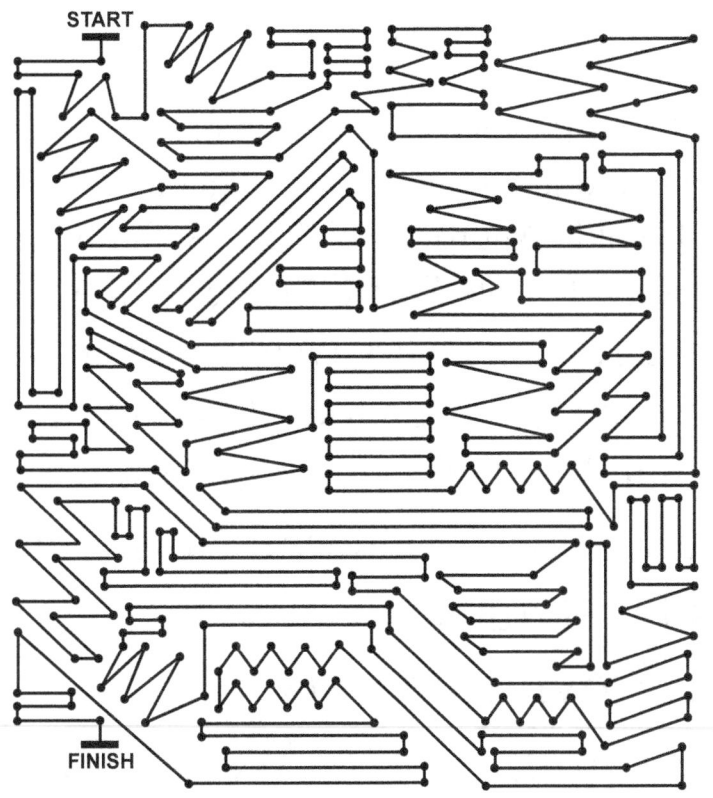

Acuity Chart

Palace Hotel Book Genuine Perfume Insight Movie Airplane Show Heaven Good Hold Twinkle Command Manning Teach Bold Peace Nurse Family Zoo Donate Therapy Hug Develpe Pretty Admire Honey Foot Capacity Listen Wealthy Musk Loving Extra Big Jungle Mountains Babysitting Playroom Above Yelling Queue Pencil Rotate Arms •03

Finish Mood Velvet Orange Crayons Gum Desk Magic Time Regular Express Scholar Rainbow Decor Europe Moving Clarity Forgive Concert Weekend Guide Essentials Volume Between Log Elbow Muscle Chart White Eyesight Zone Recommend Cure Food •04

Ceiling Pants Booster Negativity Contact Lifestyle Glad Modem Tailor Marketplace Optical School Twice Supplements Fifteen Day Brush Count Mastered Blur Tango Inches Second Toxic Amount Plums Tie •05

Alternate Over Highheels Cardoor Boxes Willow Thin Smart Repeat Precription Mistakes Photocopy Delay Bumper Sideways Midnight Teeth Circumstance Voice Stimulate •06

Lenses Excuse Motivation Backwards Rotation Verbal Blink Outline Piece Eyelids Pleasantly Muscle Return Bottom Down Panel Survival Cute Try •07

Forward Organize Speakers Pound Rose Number Far Lungs Center Squeeze Forehead Tissue Safe Allow Inform Month Billboard •08

Improve Doctor Hand Thin Remember Diamond Letter Optic Survival Office Automobiles Card Motorboat Twenty •09

Woman Fur Kaleidoscope Planning Red Concentrate Beauty Deference Jack Motion Sail Illusions Often •10

Flashes View Range Sleep Duration Fatigue Elevator Several Days Helicopter Knitting Nobody •11

Yelp Afternoon Racing Eagle Monkey Please Tower Window Calendar Statue Hurrican •12

Pig Why Frozen Wrinkle Jackpot Lettuce Spiral Bounce Shop Up Triangle Small •13

Future Nails Top Cupcakes Powerful Vision Tomorrow Sunset Connections •14

Black Keyboard Handbag Numbers Watch Booze Candy Plug Internet •15

Quality Charcter Jumping Rod Book Party Lightning Cereal Fend •16

Plant Strong Purify Vent Duke Butterfly Kingdom Cellphones •17

Makeup Theater Rabbit Cup Extend Letter Closed Dancer •18

You Singing Explain Fond Zoom Judgement Wonderful •19

Genuine Twinkle Android Chickens Ballet Neverland •20

Fun Education People World Music Yelling Ranger •21

Excite Long Roman Doors Weather Open Silence •22

Allow Serene Humor Lagoon Takeout Musk Be •23

Village Snug Kitchen Love Amazingly Giving •24

Protecting Change Wonderful Noise Summer •25

Holidays Fund Sunshine Vow American No •26

Next Like Provide Important Mow English •27

Sow Listen Jump Honey Wealth Powerful •28

Myself Elephant Conquer Puppy Follow •29

We Maybe Admire Computer Glass Joy •30

Serene Flowing Angle Survive Perfect •31

Nose Paradise Key Worship Together •32

References

1   What's in a Cigarette? American Lung Association. Accessed at: http://www.lung.org/stop-smoking/about-smoking/facts-figures/whats-in-a-cigarette.html

2   J Levenson et al., "Cigarette Smoking and Hypertension," Arteriosclerosis 7 (1987): 572-7.

3   H Kritz, P Schmid and H Sinzinger, "Passive Smoking and Cardiovascular Risk," Arch Intern Med 155 (1995): 1942-8.